Overcoming the Deadly Depression

Holistic approaches to

depression and anxiety therapy

Sam Oluwaseyi

TABLE OF CONTENTS

OVERCOMING THE DEADLY DEPRESSION I

INTRODUCTION 6

THE RICH ALSO CRY 6

CHAPTER 1 17

WHAT IS DEPRESSION? 17

CHAPTER 2 29

SYMPTOMS OF DEPRESSION 29

CHAPTER 3 41

CAUSES OF DEPRESSION 41

CHAPTER 4 75

TYPES OF DEPRESSION 75

CHAPTER 5 91

OVERCOMING THE DEADLY DEPRESSION 91

CHAPTER 6 100

WHEN YOU NEED A PSYCHRIATRIST 100

CHAPTER 7 110

APPROACHES TO TREATMENT OF DEPRESSION......................110

CHAPTER 8 124

PHARMACOLOGY APPROACH TO TREATMENT OF DEPRESSION 124

CHAPTER 9 144

ALTERNATIVE THERAPIES 144

CHAPTER 10 155

FAITH BASED APPROACH TO TREATMENT OF DEPRESSION........................155

ABOUT THE AUTHOR **185**

ACKNOWLEDGMENTS **186**

Holistic Approaches to Depression and Anxiety Therapy

ABOUT THE AUTHOR **185**

ACKNOWLEDGMENTS **186**

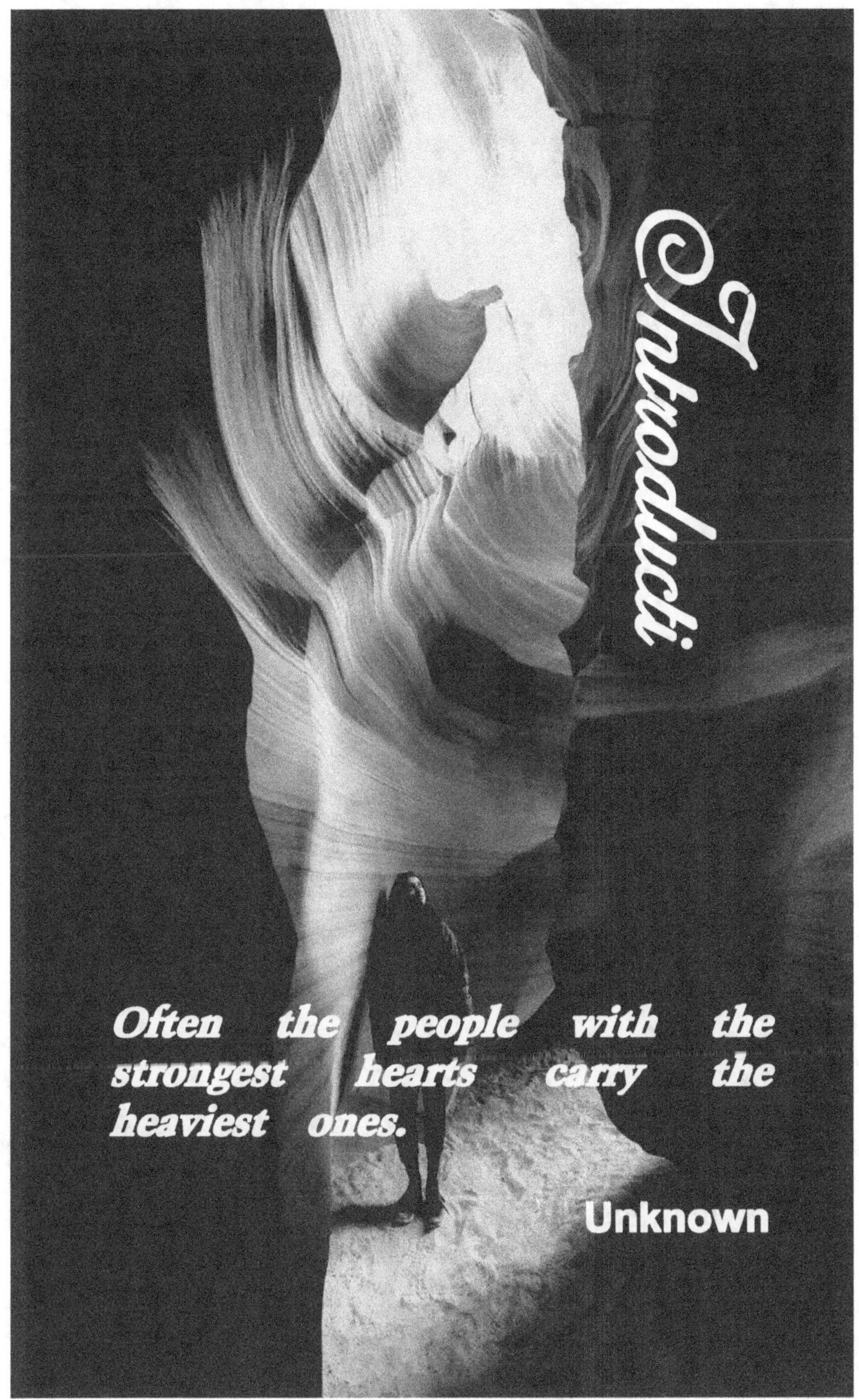
Introducti

Often the people with the strongest hearts carry the heaviest ones.

Unknown

Introduction

THE RICH ALSO CRY

Someone has once described the universe as a chaotic space where all manner of uneventful happens. You wake up in the morning to start up your day but you possibly don't know what may happen the next hour.

All-day along, we come across people who look nice, wear great perfumes; everywhere are people who wear all manner of looks on their faces. Some, nice to behold theirs while many go about painting their sorrows on their faces.

Life may be funny at times. In it is all manner of events, good and bad, nice and distasteful, sweet and sour, smiles and aggression, merriment and melancholy, elevation and demotion/job termination, fruitiness and barrenness, and the list goes on. Where do all these events happen? The answer is simple, yes, they happen in the minds of humans. Sometimes, we let these events define who we are and how

people perceive us, this often forms the basis for how they relate with us.

Humans are likened to containers; these containers come with different sizes. The amount of weight one can contain differs from another. Some times in life, we enjoy the memories of life when it is a good thing that always comes across our ways, this may be a thing we may never have to be bothered about because they give us joy.

On the other hand, when life comes with its ugly side, we seem to struggle to stay focus and be in charge. These chaotic moments come around, we seem to be bothered about these situations and try to maintain focus with our normal life; we drop our supposed worries, failure, fear of the unknown etc in the container. As life challenges mount, we keep piling them up in the container and the process continues. Even a simple challenge that could have been remedied earlier is thrown in the container.

At a point in time, the container gets overwhelmed and has no more space to contain the garbage any longer. There are struggles to retain the old garbage while new ones keep coming.

Your mind is like the container filled with different forms of life disappointments, worries, fears, etc. overtime piled in our minds, and we are often on the disadvantage. Anxiety, fear of the unknown, memories of our failure, molestation among others keep hurting us, thus, making man helpless. There is an alarming increase in the rate of suicide in the world. The aforementioned could be responsible.

These negative life events which may be unforgiveness, loneliness, hopelessness, failure in a life pursuit, bad marital experience; disappointment from a lover who you have planned your life with, or worst, someone who you have given up all you have unto disappear into the thin air, marital infidelity from your spouse, rejections from members of your family, or you just been fired at your place of work for no moral reasons; molestation from close allies, death of a wife having a baby behind, the list are endless, bring bitterness and sorrow to someone's life.

Depression is a genuine mental issue facing a consistently expanding number of people in our contemporary society. It is often called the common cold of mental illness, psychological sickness among other names. It affects individuals from all works of life and irrespective of their status in society.

Did I hear you asked, "You mean the rich? " Yes, the rich, "the rich likewise cry". I have seen a rich person who parked his car on a highway and jumped into a river. That was his end.

Religious leaders are not exempted either from the ugly effects of depression.

Many you look up to as social role models are not left out of depression. Yes, many you call successful in the field of athletics, wrestling, boxing, football, sports generally, will tell you the level of depression they had had to contend with.

A friend shares an interesting story of a depressive Neil. The experience of Neil may inspire you. He said that depression could happen to a person who always goes about wearing a smiling face, a jovial person telling jokes and fun to always be with, "which I am'.

For Neil, one would wonder why he could experience depression alluding to the fact that he has a family, a good and to say the least, he is okay.

"So why may I be depressed? For Neil said It was hard for him to speak to people because he was not sure what their reactions would be towards him. "Previously, I've realized that individuals were talking behind me, disclosing to me that they required assistance, but 'I am also "poor", they didn't know.

But the ironical part of it is that the rich also cry and need a shoulder to lean on. This was so in Neil because he found himself as the one who is the needy, at least, "I also needed someone who I can lean on," he said.

He said when you have been that figure of respect, love and inspirations to others, giving advice or counselling people of good living, and suddenly the roles turn around and you find yourself been on the receiving end.

Sometimes, one might consider it okay to die in silence while the societal respects go on because humans can be so hasty to judge. That alone is depressing.

He said, "it is either I put on these masks and wear a smiling face, pushing everything back…or I become perplexed. There appears to be 'no one in-between as I found it difficult to see someone who I could talk to. I don't know how to speak. My feelings have affected my own private life because rather, I react with "a fight or flight". I either need to scream and shout how tough my experience is, or I just want to run and cover which is not good to the people I love.

And there comes the confusing or screaming voices inside that brings about perplexity. Even when doing your normal tasks in your house or selecting what to, Neil felt like that was an explosion in his head because he was struggling to stay focused. "Because I cannot figure out what goes on within me. So this is when my "fight or flight" kicks in," He added.

Neil attests to the fact that this mood changes with time and come again, "Thankfully this is not all the time and greatly relies upon on how I am feeling that day, as I even have my best days and terrible days too. Some days I am as glad as I can be like nothing is wrong, however, this may change so quickly. For me, I need to open up to someone, let people in and learn to talk but I also believe we need to stay in an atmosphere where the judgment is left out and depression is acknowledged, and we can openly talk," Neil said.

You may be shocked and asked, then who is free from depression? Don't get it wrong, the purpose of this book is not to magnify the existence of the problem, depression, but to face the problem itself while vigorous and holistic approaches are employed to proffer solutions to the phenomenon, depression.

Depression imposes itself not only on adults but it takes its toll on children and adolescents as well. This may seem true, in the words of Bo Burnham, an American Comedian and poet who said, "Once a week, I like to slip into a deep existential depression where I lose all my sense of oneness and self-worth".

"Often the people with the strongest hearts carry the heaviest ones".

Unknown

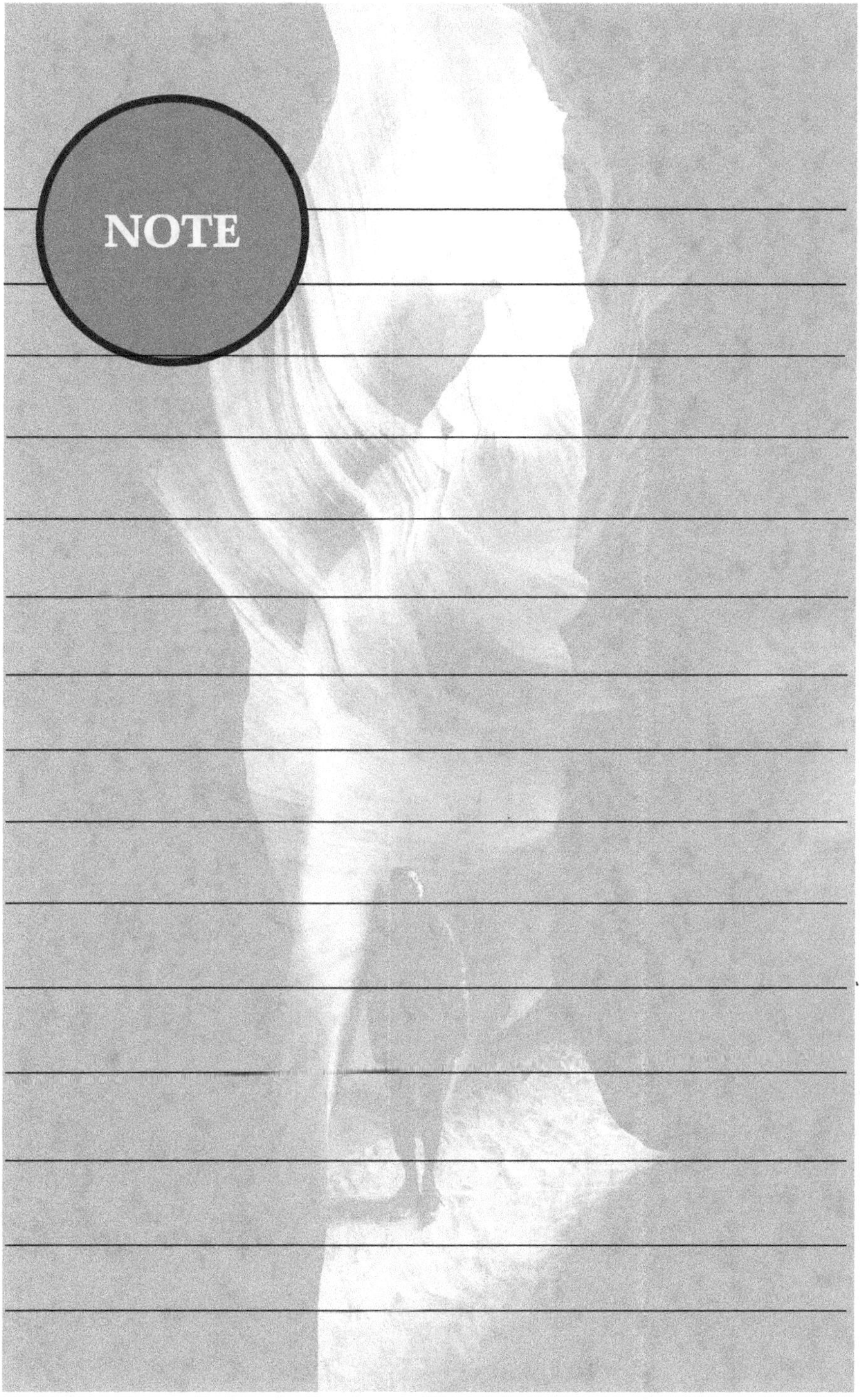

NOTE

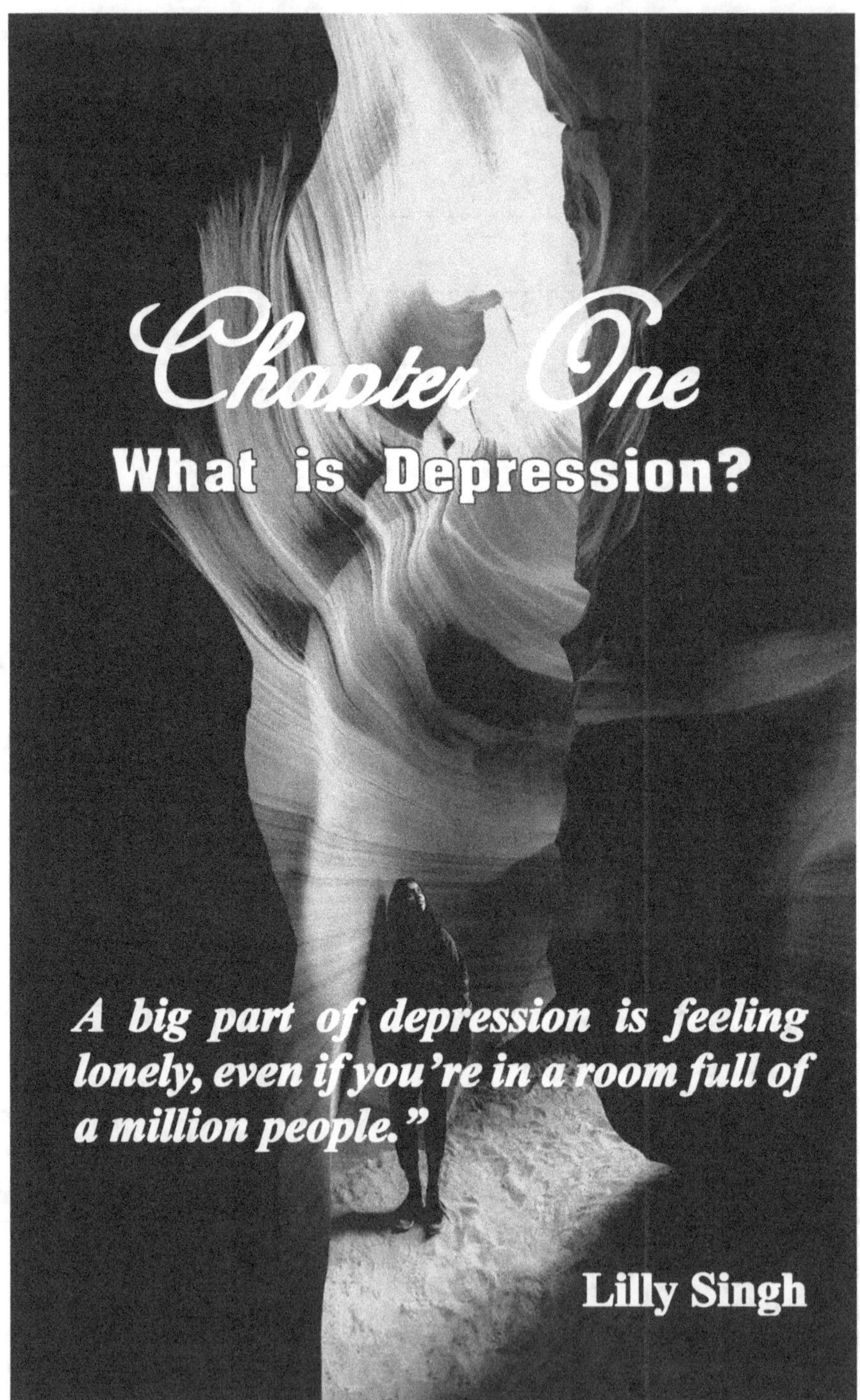
Chapter One
What is Depression?
A big part of depression is feeling lonely, even if you're in a room full of a million people."
Lilly Singh

Chapter 1

What is Depression?

Depression is a general and severe health condition that affects how someone feels, thinks and acts daily. Depression can be capable of interfering with routine functioning of the human mind, and regularly causing complications with work, social and family adjustment.

Depression brings various degrees of devastating experiences, meaninglessness to life, hopelessness, obscurity, among others, to a person. It is said to be a 'silent killer', which makes a person go about as a 'living sepulchre'.

Depression will be the best delineated as a combination of physical and mental symptoms. And each of those kinds of symptoms can decrease the activity and performance of the brain. A person affected by depression will experience multiple symptoms like disappointment, cynicism, irritability, and absence of specializing in everyday activities, inferiority complex, sluggish digestion etc. It could be a grave disorder that produces the sufferer incapable of operating as well as collaborating in day to day activities. It could be a condition that causes simply restricted annoyance in the day to day life.

Depression, according to World Health Organization (WHO), defines it as a sickness characterized by unhappiness, loss of interest or pleasure, emotions of guilt or low self-worth, disordered sleep or craving, attenuated strength and terrible concentration.

It all depends, depression may be periodical, typically which comes and goes. However, its life cycle maybe with some sorts driven via genetic, biological factors and other kinds being an extra response to most important life events.

The depressed persons may easily become so uninteresting, passive and unsympathetic about personal hygiene, eating habits, among other activities; that the patients may require an increased amount of time to execute their daily chores,"

World Health Organization said depression is a common mental disorder. Worldwide, about 264 million individuals of all ages suffer from depression. Depression may be a leading reason behind incapacity worldwide and is a major contributor to the international burden of illness. It often results in suicide. There are viable mental and pharmacological treatments for both moderate and severe depression. The WHO said women are more affected by depression than men.

Depression may be a common malady worldwide, with over 264 million individuals affected. Depression is completely different from usual mood fluctuations and fugacious emotional responses to challenges in daily life, particularly once lasting and with moderate or severe intensity, depression could become a heavy health condition. It will cause the affected person to suffer greatly and perform poorly at work, at college and within the family. It can lead to a situation whereby the sufferer gets rid of his/her life. Around 800,000 individuals pass on yearly because of suicide. Globally, records have it that suicide is the predominant cause of death among people between 15-29-years-old.

Many aged depressed persons are mistaken for individuals with dementedness due to their concentration is thus impaired that it looks their memory has weakened. The person may become psychotic, hearing voices or believing things that aren't leading staff to think them as schizophrenic.

Agitated depression may come with an increased form of irritability, brooding, pacing, and distress; it produces several issues for the employees and alternative residents. The person could become either frightened by a spoken word or physically.

Worldwide, records have it that over 264 million people are affected by depression. It is different in relation to routine mood changes and short-lived emotional reactions to challenges in regular daily life. Above all as long-lasting and with moderate or vigorous intensity, depression may suit a dangerous health condition. It can bring about the artificial guise to be diagnosed with exceedingly and event poorly at work, at work and in the family. At its worst, depression can lead to suicide in the end. Suicide is the second chief source of mortality in 15-29-years-old, and the second cause of disability in the world, according to the WHO report.

Records give insights; state that it's in most extraordinary cases, it can prompt suicide, representing around 850,000 fatalities every year. In the United States alone, the most common form of depression and mental disorder in the

Major Depressive Disorder (MDD), is diagnosed when a severely depressed mood and activity level that persists for two weeks or more and affected 6.4% of the

U.S. adult population in 2008. It is the main individual illness (disease) or disorder in the US and Canada.

The National Institute of Mental Health (NIMH) reports that in disability- lost due to illness, disability, and sudden death, more than ischemic heart disease, liquor (alcohol) use issue, or pulmonary years.

In Africa, depression has great effects on the continent with depressive disorder and dysthymia; having similar symptoms. Dysthymia is believed to be chronic and lasts for longer than the depressive disorder. A recent report from Global Health via the World Health Organization, Says base on the numbers of people tested, having in mind that, but not all the people with depressive disorders, says many components affect the rate of diagnosis, including mental health awareness and the availability of psychiatric facilities. Djibouti, Cape

Verde and Tunisia, Lesotho, Botswana, Ethiopia, Uganda and South Africa, being the first-seven top depressed nations in Africa, Djibouti tops the list with 5.1% of its population suffering from depressive disorders, the country is adjudged Africa's most depressed country.

In Europe, the WHO says, "Each year, 25% of the population suffers from depression or anxiety." Neuropsychiatric disorders account for 19.5% of the burden of disease in the European Region, and 26% in the European Union (EU) countries.

These disorders represent up to 40% of years lived with disability, with depression as the primary cause.

About half (50%) of major depressions are not treated.

The expense of mood of disorder and anxiety in the EU is about €170 billion every year.

Are the young ones left out of depression? No! It is as predominant among children as well as teenagers. We all want necessities for them and make them safe, but despite parents doing their best to provide and protection and guidance to their children, they may still be a disappointment, frustrated, or heartbroken. Sometimes, they feel miserable and needy. However, some children and adolescents seem to be constantly experiencing sorrow, hopelessness, and helplessness. Depression is an illness where the feelings of despondence persist and intervene with the child or adolescent functional ability. Depression is not always manifested by the sadness in adolescents but by irritability, boredom, or ineptitude to feel pleasure. Depression is a chronic, recurrent, and mostly an inherited illness. Frequently, the first appearance of depression occurs during childhood or adolescence. Prolonged depressive situations happen in an individual with dysthymic disorder, gradually progresses into major depression.

Depression in teenagers is a disabling situation that is connected with meaningful extensive stretch morbidity and suicide consistently. American Academy of Child and Adolescent Psychiatry (AACAP), said about five per cent of the all children population may experience depression at any time and that fact keeps rising.

"Often the people with the strongest hearts carry the heaviest ones."

Unknown.

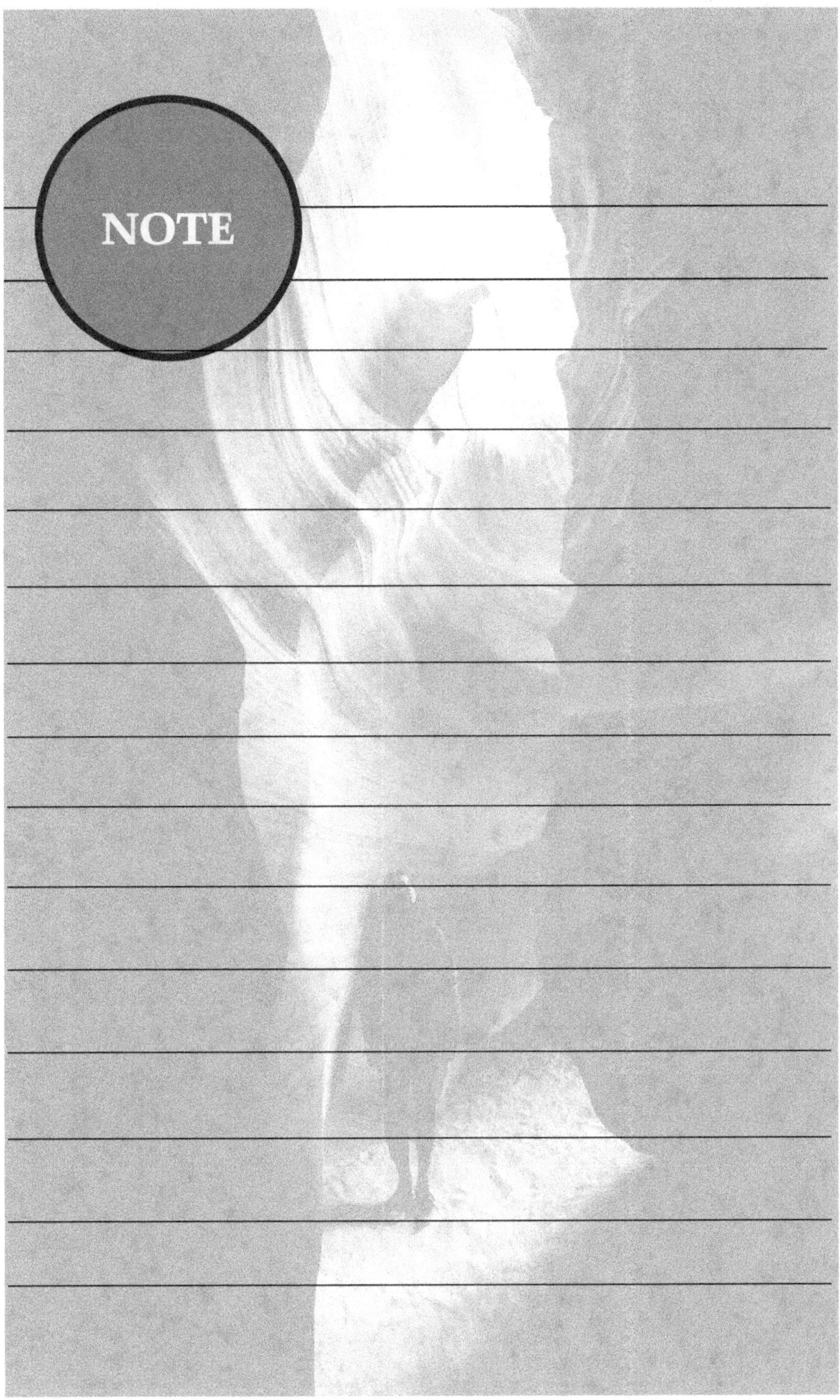
NOTE

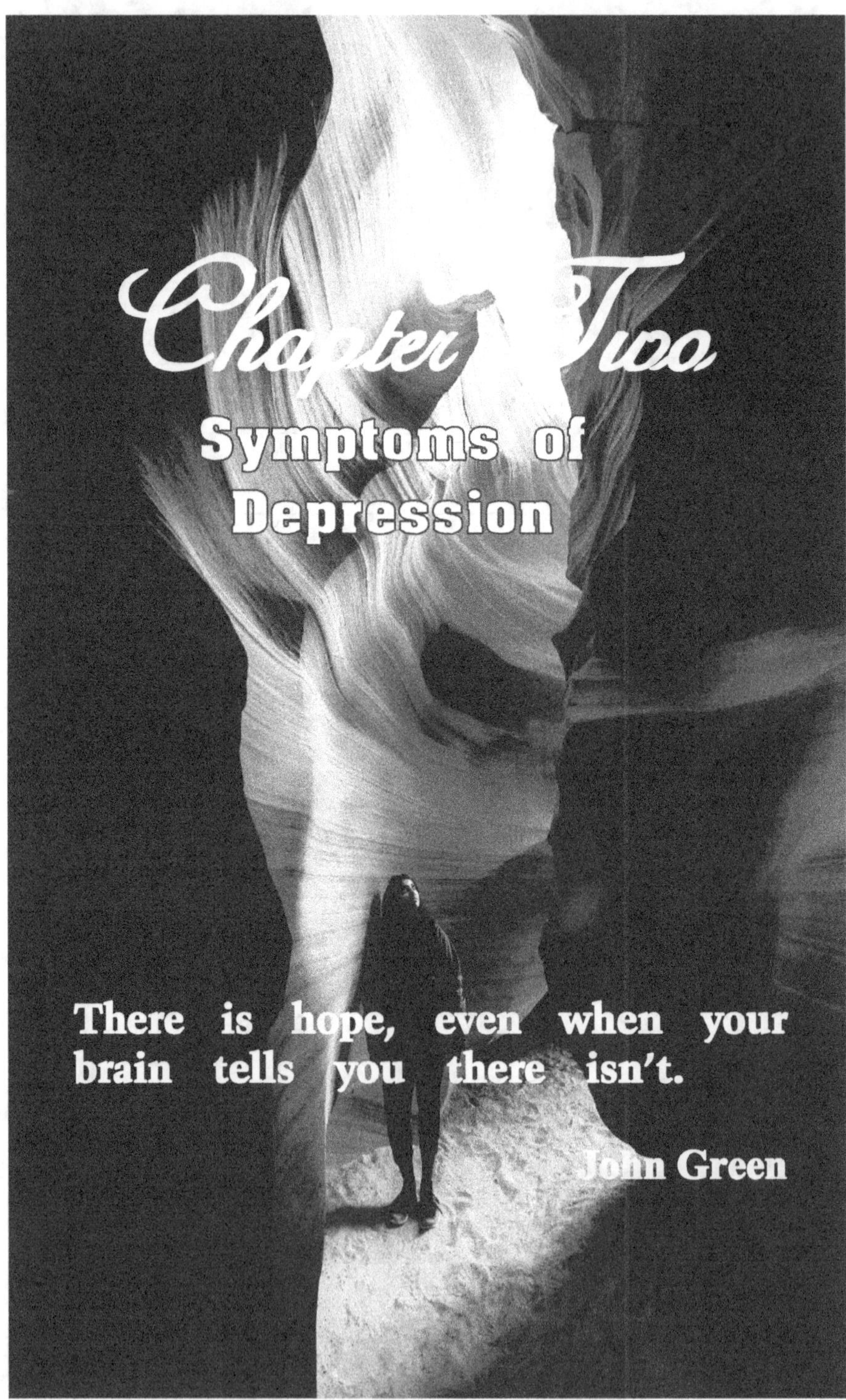
Chapter Two
Symptoms of Depression
There is hope, even when your brain tells you there isn't.
John Green

Chapter 2

SYMPTOMS OF DEPRESSION

The feeling of unhappiness is a normal response to everyday disagreeable,disappointing or displeasing eve nts like losing a beloved or running into monetary problem or rejection from loved ones. Depression can easily be identified by tracking some of the common symptoms. It could be as a result of bad moods and things around which may seem wrong to the person experiencing depression while having in mind difficulty people feel in sleeping and waking. These could be insomnia, nightmare sleep, oversleeping and among others.

On a general note, depression symptoms can come in different forms, it can be feelings of sadness or unhappiness. The irony of unhappiness is that the sufferer may even be in the entertainment industry, making people cast away their boredoms, yet languishing in depression. Frustration or irritability is another general symptom of depression, the sufferer oftentimes gives up easily. Their hope and endurance systems seem disturbed which may bring loss of interest or pleasure in normal activities that give bring about relaxation.

A depressed person once said anytime time he had sex with his wife, he struggled to satisfy her, the reason given is that I get a lot of loads in my chest (mind) that just don't let me concentrate. Another said I stay without the feeling of sex for weeks. They're lost for sex drive is said to be likened to someone in a fully air-conditioned room but wetting profusely. Sleeplessness (insomnia) or excessive sleeping, loss of appetite and weight, but in some people the reverse can be the case whereby there would be cravings for food and weight gain. Agitation or restlessness which could be angry outbursts, disruptive or reckless behaviour, complexity in sitting still, wringing the hands or cleaning the fists, problems with focusing or having a conversation.

Symptoms will seem suddenly or overtime. They will additionally vary from a shrewish sense of unease to aggression. If agitation results in impulsive or aggressive behaviour, it might lead to damage to the person or others.

Some other general symptoms of depression:

- Slowed speaking, body movement or thinking indecisiveness, distractibility and decreased attention

- Distraction, Indecisiveness, and decreased concentration

- fatigue, tiredness and lack of energy even in small obligations might also seem to require a whole lot of effort

- emotions of worthlessness or guilt, obsession on past failures or blaming yourself whilst matters are not going right

- trouble in thinking, concentrating, making decisions and remembering matters or things.

- Frequent thoughts of death, dying or suicide

- Crying spells for no obvious reasons

- Unexplained bodily problems, e.g backaches or headaches.

Depression symptoms in children and teenagers

The symptoms of depression in children and teenager can be quite different from it seems in adults. It may be a sign of sadness, hopelessness, worry, and irritability. It may also be a sense of avoidance of social life or interaction (children may frequently withdraw from social activities in the presence of their peer. Lack of social interactions in children may cause social fear and anxiety or be lonely), anger or anxiety.

Depression may bring about changes in sleeping and thinking of the sufferer, this is not a sign that often in younger children. Mental health and behavioural problems in children and teens include several types of emotional and behavioural disorders, including disruptive, depression, anxiety and pervasive developmental (autism) disorders, characterized as either internalizing or externalizing problems. Disruptive activity issues like temper tantrums, attention-deficit upset disorder, oppositional, intractable or conduct disorders are the most common issues in the commonest behavioural problems in teens and young children.

Children with depression may suffer concentration in schoolwork. My personal experience as an instructor corroborates this. An encounter with one of my students, a girl, who came to me for counselling, said that she was easily carried away from class activity. The funny part was when she said some male instructors, to her, often look like some who have physically molested before.

She said, I can't concentrate, there is no amount of whacking or punishments that can make me understand anything." It was then I realized that another approach was needed to be applied in teaching her.

Other symptoms of depression in adolescents can be any of the following:

- Depressed or irritable mood.

- Temper, agitation.

- lack of interest and decreased gratification in daily activities.

- Change in appetite, usually a loss of appetite.

- Persistent difficulty falling asleep or staying asleep (insomnia).

- Sleeping difficulty.

- Excessive daytime sleepiness or general fatigue.

- Difficulty concentrating and memory loss.

- Preoccupation with self.

- attitudes of worthlessness or disappointment.

- Excessive or inappropriate guilt feelings.

- Acting out behaviour.

- Thoughts about suicide or abnormal thoughts about death.

- Thought to commit suicide or attempt suicide attempt.

- An excessively irresponsible behaviour pattern.

Depression symptoms in older adults

The signs of depression in adults may be:

In older adults, depression may go undiagnosed because symptoms, for instance, loss of appetite, tiredness, sleep problems or loss of interest in sex may seem to be caused by other illnesses.

older adults with depression may additionally have less noticeable symptoms. they may have a sense of disappointments with life, in general, they may also feel bored, helpless or worthless. they'll continually need to live at home, instead of going out to socialise or doing new things.

suicidal thoughts or emotions in older adults is an indication of great despair that have to never be taken gently, especially in men. Of everybody with depression, the older person (men) are at the highest risk of suicide.

From the above, it is evident that there are various symptoms of depression. It will be very wrong for someone to hastily generalize a treatment for depression without first knowing the cause. But the truth is that whichever symptoms of depression you may have, following and knowing the kind of trend or form of depression manifesting in you will go a long way to understand the best type of treatment for you.

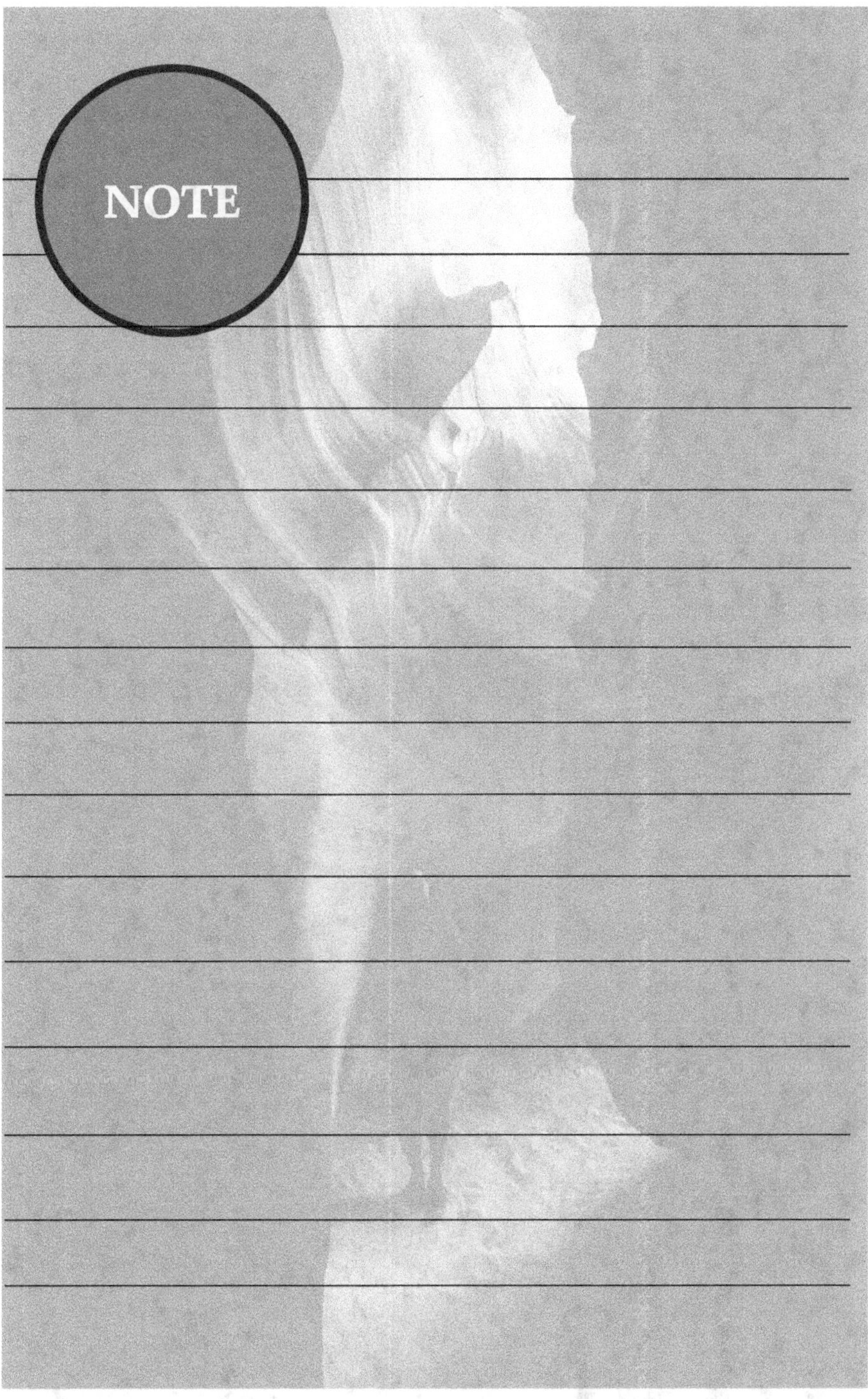

NOTE

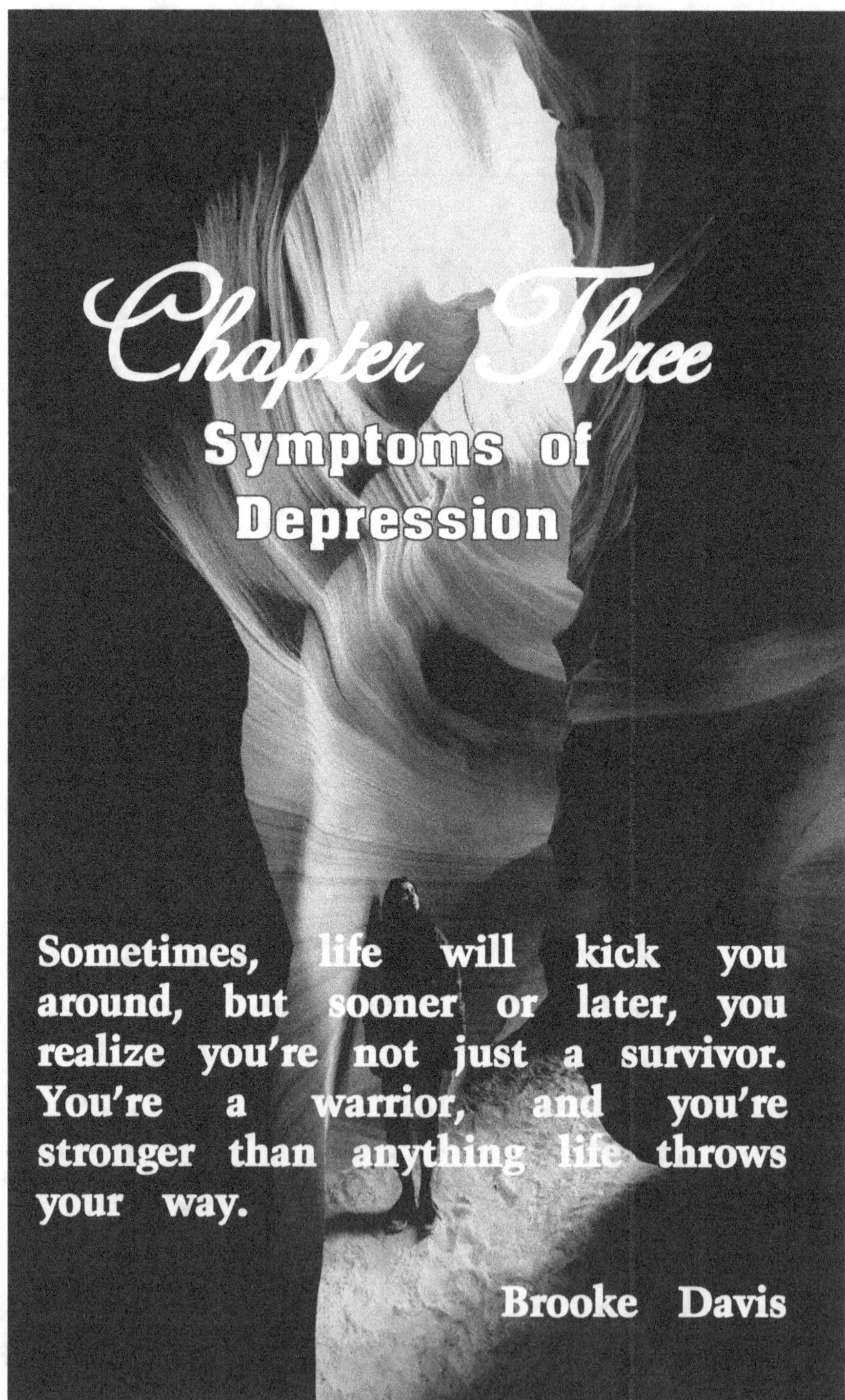
Chapter Three
Symptoms of
Depression

Sometimes, life will kick you
around, but sooner or later, you
realize you're not just a survivor.
You're a warrior, and you're
stronger than anything life throws
your way.

Brooke Davis

Chapter 3

CAUSES OF DEPRESSION

Next chapter gives elaborate details on the types of depression. Depression is a complex whole. No one can boldly tell the real cause of depression because the symptoms of depression differ from one person to another. A young lady may experience depression during menstruation, while for another; it may be a serious medical illness. Economy situation of a country may be responsible to some people's depression. Accounts of these abound in many third-world countries. The relocation or death of a loved one can also cause depression among other cause.

Genetic factors

You are at a higher risk of developing depression if you have a family history of depression or other kinds mood disorder. Family and twin studies show that genetic factor is a high potential of having depression. "Twin research data shows that the heritability rate for depression is 37% (95% CI: 31%–42%), and data from family studies show a two-to-threefold increase in the risk of depression in first-degree offspring of patients with depression." Similarly, studies have shown that those having relatives with depression experience stand the risk of developing similar problem. A Director of Health, Cedars-Sinai Medical Center in Los Angeles, Lekeisha A. Summer, said that individuals with siblings or parents having Major Depression have approximately two to three times higher familiar risk and that the risk is even worse …"

In a family study underwent, the result showed that relatives of depressed children have higher rate of major depressive disorder (MDD) compared to the relatives of healthy children. Research shows that individuals with folks or siblings who have depression are up to a few times more probably going to possess the condition. Hereditary factor is seen to have a robust influence on circumstance. However, it is not too clear if psychiatric ailment so have immediate effects on members of a family who suffers metal ailment.

A recent research carried out by British researchers isolated a gene that seems to be prevailing in multiple members of the family with depression. The chromosome 3p25-26 was found in more than 800 families with intermittent depression.

Having established that depression can be hereditary. A study which was carried out on several generations of families who at a point in time had survived a devastating earthquake in Asian country; researchers discovered that about 60% of depressive episodes when the event happened had a genetic link. This study suggests that our DNA plays a minimum of some role in raising the chance for depression. Scientists are simply commencing to uncover the explanations behind that genetic link.

A study published in the journal Neuron revealed that, "one specific gene, SLC6A15, may factor into determining which people are at an increased risk of depression. Their work suggests that when this specific gene is shortened, it alters the brain's ability to carry chemical messages. The modified gene may also harm the integrity of neurons, which are specialized nerve cells," Ranch Treatment Center, 2020. Researchers are hopeful this sort of genetic finding will cause targeted antidepressants at intervals successive ten to fifteen years.

Recent psychological health (mental health) analysis posits that people living with depression tend to possess smaller hippocampus functionality in the brain – than those who don't suffer the disorder. The hippocampus plays an important role in someone's emotion or feeling, memory and learning.

ascertain is whether or not having a smaller hippocampus triggers depression, or whether or not the upper levels of stress hormones in depressed individuals shrinks that a part of the brain. What's clear is that depression could be a complicated mental disorder which will solely be absolutely understood with the assistance of progress analysis.

Truly depression runs in families. However, by being proactive you'll be able to cut back your risk of developing the disorder or keep the symptoms to a bearest minimum if they are doing occur. It is never ahead of time to begin managing your stress and building a foundation for a good permanent psychological health condition.

Environmental factor

Environment is defined as the complex of physical, chemical, and biotic factors (such as climate, soil, and living things) that act upon an organism or an ecological community and ultimately determine its form and survival; the aggregate of social and cultural conditions that influence the life of an individual or community.

Environmental factor also contribute to depression which are present around us, they may be in form of air, water and nutritional pollution. Noise is a non-chemical source of environmental stress. Other non-chemical pollutions include electrical pollution, natural disasters, and other catastrophic environmental events.

Studies are still being carried out to ascertain the precise relationship between environmental factors and depression. It is a known fact that air and water pollution would have physiological consequences like cancer and birth defects.

There is a belief system that pollution in our environment has great influence on our mental health. For instance, "sick building syndrome" is a condition caused by exposure to numerous corrupting agents in a very "sick building," sometimes associate workplace or different building that homes many folks operating in short proximity between a person to another. People with sick building syndrome tend to become terribly anxious and irritable; they will hyperventilate and develop intermittent cramp and/or severe shortness of breath.

Some natural events in life which take place in our environments have a great deal of effect in our emotions. Natural disasters like hurricanes, tsunamis, and earthquakes, will contribute to an already vulnerable person's status to depression. These aforementioned environmental factors may bring the tendency to become depressed. Such sufferer may also develop symptoms after they encounter significant and traumatic environmental situations.

Environment factor has causative effects on adolescents. Parenting behaviors and family environment are same to possess a large influence in child's adaptation throughout the vital years. With successful adaptation, to the youngster's environment, such is ready for future development challenges.

Another factor that has a significant impact over children's rising view of themselves is the educational system, the school. The current self-framework during youth and teenagers can be sustained especially by school settings (that incorporates school climate, educator and peer relations, and scholarly disappointment in school works or underachievement) that give open doors for help, self-governance and relatedness.

Kids figure out how to see themselves from how others see them. On the off chance that they are reliably feed with negative recognitions or perception, which ordinarily happen to youngsters with lower academic performance, such children would in the end see themselves as incapable. The child's negative self-recognition can add to the improvement of depressive attitudes.

Studies found consistent evidences that educational issues are often the organic process pathway to depressive symptoms throughout childhood. That claim may still need to be proven further. A youngster, who is frequently the object of harassing or bullying, is liable to peer dismissal and low confidence. Negative sentiments came about because of harassing can turn into a grapple of negative feelings, for example, sorrow, tension, dejection, and insecurity.

To certain kids, incessant harassing and bullying prompt dangerous results. There is relationship between bully victimization and suicidal thoughts tendency in a child in such situation.

Depression can often be triggered by very stressful life situations or other factors in our environment.

Psychological Factors

Psychological factors put a lot of people at risk of depression. Life situations such as lost of a loved one, low self-esteem, lost of job, failure, marital malady, among other negative events in life. Those affected often see life with pessimism and are more overwhelmed by stress which eventually leads to depression.

Cognitive disturbances occur in depression. A cognitive disturbances patient develops a pessimistic view of himself and interprets the experiences negatively by misperceiving the situations.

In a case of loss of a loved one, depressed patients often have ambivalent feelings towards their loved ones. This hostility when depressed from consciousness leads to depression.

A basic model of mind comprising id., ego and superego, stressed that in depressed people there is a pulling back of libidinal connection from the lost object which is for the most part put resources into an individual's own ego as opposed to in another item. The piece of this libidinal energy served to set up a recognizable proof of the sense of ego with the neglected object: while the rest of the libido gets a twisted essentially the struggle between ego and superego replaces struggle between ego and the complicatedly adored object extended the idea of introjections. Thus, concluding that depressed patients normally look on certain physical and mental attributes of the late friends or family member(s).

By using this framework of structural theory of mind, it suggested that in depressed patients the hostile impulses which originated from id come into conflict with the ego and the rigid punitive superego, and thus resulted in feelings of guilt and depression.

Another study showed that during the first year of child's life, kid builds up a relationship with his mother; children respond to dissatisfaction and frustrations with rage and cruel motivations. Until the child can come to understanding of being cherished in spite of his anger, each dissatisfaction is deciphered by the baby as lost the great object or the good mother. The feelings of this misery, blame and lament that go with this apparent object misfortune are known as depressive state. She further inferred that kids who feel lacking in affection during the depressive position are inclined to repeated assaults of depressive assaults when they grow up into adult life.

The theory of learned helplessness described depressives as incompetent individuals who fail to handle the aversive life situations and hence give up things easily. Other behaviourists believed that in depression there is a failure to receive positive reinforcement which leads to reduction in the activities, thus results in less chances of coping with these situations and needs gratification by becoming ill.

The psychological hereditary impact of depression is the same in adolescents. Young people who saw their parents or guardians to have moderately equivalent power or fathers to have more power than mothers are said to be preferred and have both social and emotional results than teenagers who revealed that their mother had more power than their fathers. The study submitted that adherence to socially recommended roles and standards of spousal relationships are probably going to bring about the most alluring arrangement of child's results.

Young people who are depressed have more negative impression of their families than others do. The more depressed the youngster, the more negative are his views of the manner by which his family functions. In particular, depressed young people portray their parents as far off, unsupportive, and emotionally detached from them.

These depressed children often consider their parents to be as narrow minded, firm and intolerable. They feel that they don't feel relevant in matters that affect the family. They lack the basic courage to withstand live challenges. Like a saying has it, "Charity begins at home." Conclusively, depressed adolescents report that their families hardly have bonding time together in as families in social, religious, or recreational exercises. Compared to parents and guardians of non-depressed children, parents of depressed children are increasingly dictator and control their interactions with their children.

Sociocultural Factors

Sociocultural factors reliably have been perceived as major factor in connoting the unconventionality in the commonness of depression, mostly in older people. With the progression in modernization, instances of physical and mental well-being issues are expanding continuously and society become mechanical. The desire of popularity and money makes an individual denied of sociocultural values. Along these lines, older people are altogether influenced by medical problems including melancholy. Also, stress full life occasions, obliviousness from relatives, loss of friends and family member, financial emergencies, period of retirement, and both inter and intra-personal clashes went with other medical problems lead to late life.

Also social factors seem to play an important role in the onset, course, and outcome of depressive disorders. These factors such as social class, migration, urbanization, and family conditions have been shown to be associated with psychiatric syndromes such as schizophrenia, manic-depressive psychosis, and other neurotic disorders.

Studies in psychiatry, showed that first admissions for schizophrenia were more prevalent in poor, socially disorganized, overcrowded and the central areas of the cities while for manic-depressive psychosis these were random. Similar studies were carried out in other American Cities and in Norway.

Earlier studies have shown that there is a close association between psychiatric illnesses mainly schizophrenia with low social status, whereas for depressive psychosis it was found evenly distributed. In some studies it was found that the referral rates for all mental illnesses were higher from sodal class I and II (professionals and managerials), while other studies reported these rates from Class V; and for depression the higher rates were found in class III i.e. skilled and non-manual workers.

In transcultural psychiatry, studies have shown that the incidence of these disorders varies from culture to culture. A report shows a fairly high incidence of mania in American natives, whereas depressive reactions were found relatively rare. On the contrary a totally opposite trend was found in the United States. The results were explained with respect to social values, increasing pace} and complexity of modern civilization which are the contributory factors in urban areas. Whereas, the more intimate social contacts in small communities were probable deterrents of depression in rural sample.

Advocacy on social media against the promotion of suicidal stories on the front pages of their publications as the screaming headline is a work being well done. Although more studies still need to be done on this. But what seems to be factual is that most suicide incidents that do happen mostly serve as encouragement to an individual who is depressed, thus, becoming a trend.

There are many social factors which influence either directly or indirectly the psychiatric morbidity and are considered the contributory factors. However, the presence of high degree of social support has shown to have a buffering effect against the impact of mental illness.

Peer factors

During adolescence, peers play a large part in a young person's life and typically replace the family as the centre of an adolescent's social and leisure activities. Adolescence, a child's physiological, emotional and hormonal processes come together to achieve one thing; independence from his family.

Because many children are from single-parent homes or homes in which both parents work, the amount of time adolescents spend in the company of peers is greater than ever. Negative impacts are associated with peer rejection. Rejected children are reported more loneliness, aggressive and have higher levels of depression.

Adolescents who lack friendships or have difficulty with peer relationships miss out on their many benefits.

Friends provide companionship and support each other in times of stress, such as during a parental divorce or when they are having trouble at school. Because peer relationships benefit adolescents immensely, practitioners and researchers are interested in understanding the processes by which peers reject certain children and the impact of this rejection. Some of the negative impacts associated with peer rejection are that rejected children report more loneliness and higher levels of depression than other children do.

Cliques can be a healthy part of a teen's life, but can also be dangerous to others. This was seen in the Colorado Littleton School incident in April 1999, when two senior scholars murdered 15 students as a result of their feelings of hatred towards certain groups of people at their school who had previously tormented them. The downside to cliques is that some groups are valued more highly than others and those who cannot latch into groups are somewhat disenfranchised.

Motivating factors might drive adolescents to be influenced by his friends rather than adhering to his family's ideals and values. When an adolescent feels misunderstood by his parents, he's more likely to seek out the advice, lifestyle and values of his peers.

This is challenging because it goes against parents' instincts to protect their adolescent from the risks that life presents.

Parents should not suddenly become permissive but rather that they should try to influence their adolescents not through rigid rules and strict punishment but by working to develop a good relationship with them.

When parents let their adolescents know that they respect their primary purpose; to become a unique individual, they will no longer struggle against them to achieve it.

More often than not, peers reinforce family values, but some peers, cliques and gangs have the potential to encourage problem behaviours as well.

Children today are feeling more isolated than they did in the past from the very people whom they need the most; parents, siblings and extended family members. Today, extended families are often scattered across the world. Divorced and single-parent families are prevalent, and in two-parent families, both parents often work. National statistics in America indicate that the average child sees his or her family for approximately 5-20 minutes a day. It is difficult for adolescents to feel that there is a family unit to which they belong in that short amount of time.

Consequently, this sense of isolation causes them to seek that sense of belonging elsewhere to ease the feeling of loneliness.

Creating a family "culture" will encourage children to have a sense of belonging. This family culture hinges upon parents implementing a structure that communicates in no uncertain terms to all family members that the family is more important than anything else; that the family takes priority over work, social and personal obligations.

Parents have the unique opportunity of enhancing their adolescent's self-esteem, maintaining their position as being the primary influence upon their adolescents and lessening peer influence. Influences upon a child's self-esteem as taking the shape of a pyramid with four levels. In this paradigm, a parent's unconditional love for his or her child forms the foundation of the pyramid. The second level is composed of a child's daily accomplishments. Level three involves the feedback which parents give to their children and finally, the fourth level, or top of the pyramid, is what the child's peers think about him or her. The theory is that the broader the foundation of the pyramid, the smaller the top of the pyramid is proportionally.

One way of showing unconditional love to your adolescent is by not getting sucked into the content of what she says, but instead, listening to her feelings, and developing a non-judgemental attitude, thereby keeping the lines of communication open.

Gender factors

Females are about twice as likely as males to be confirmed to have depression, this which can happen at any age in a woman's life.

Some mood changes while depression feelings happen with typical hormonal changes. In any case, hormonal changes alone don't cause depression. Other biological factors inherited traits and individual life circumstance and encounters are related with a higher chance of depression. Depression in women can also be as a result of:

Puberty: Hormone changes during puberty may increase some girls' risk of developing depression. However, temporary mood swings related to fluctuating hormones during puberty are normal. After puberty, depression rates are higher in females than in males.

Because girls typically reach puberty before boys do, they're more likely to develop depression at an earlier age than boys are. There is evidence to suggest that this depression gender gap may continue throughout the lifespan.

Premenstrual problems: For most females with premenstrual disorder (PMS), they may manifest the following symptoms, abdominal swelling, breast tenderness, headache, uneasiness, crankiness and experiencing the blues are minor and brief. It is still not clear the relationship between PMS and depression. It's conceivable that recurrent in estrogen, progesterone and some other hormones can upset the brain chemical capacity; serotonin that control mood.

Pregnancy: Hormonal changes may occur during pregnancy, and these can influence the mood of a pregnant women. Depression may increase pregnancy or during endeavors to get pregnant.

Postpartum depression: Many new mother often show depressive symptoms after child birth. Symptoms like being sad, anger and ill-tempered, and experience crying spells not long after the delivery of an offspring. These feelings some time is called baby blues. This, however, subside within a week to 14 days. But, but if continuous it can be an indication of postpartum depression.

Perimenopause and menopause: Chance of depression may increase during the progress to menopause, a phase called perimenopause, at this point, hormone levels may vacillate sporadically. Depression tendencies may likewise rise during early menopause or after menopause.

Life circumstances and culture: apart from biological reasons, depression in women may as well be caused by social reasons such as; unequal power and status, work overload, sexual or physical abuse among other social reasons.

Hard Drugs (Substance): Substance abuse: About 30% of individuals with substance abuse issues additionally have major or clinical depression. Regardless of whether these substances (drugs or liquor) briefly cause you to feel better, they at last will heighten the tendencies of being depressed.

Early childhood trauma: Tragically, parental disregard and child abuse are exceptionally common around the world. Patients mishandled or abused in adolescence, who experience neglect or the loss of a parent during childhood, are frightening experience encountered by these adolescence.

Brain structure: Studies from laboratory animal and clinical have shown impressive evidence, it indicates that stressful. Specifically, the neural and endocrine structures intervening the reaction to stress show firm alterations after childhood incidents.

Medical conditions: Serious illnesses. Sometimes depression exists together with a major illness or might be activated by another ailment.

Other risk factors for depression include:

- Low self-esteem or being self-critical

- Personal history of mental illness

- Certain medications

- Stressful events, such as loss of a loved one, economic problems, or a divorce

However, many healthcare workers are still working round the globe to unravel the puzzle put forth for the real cause of depression.

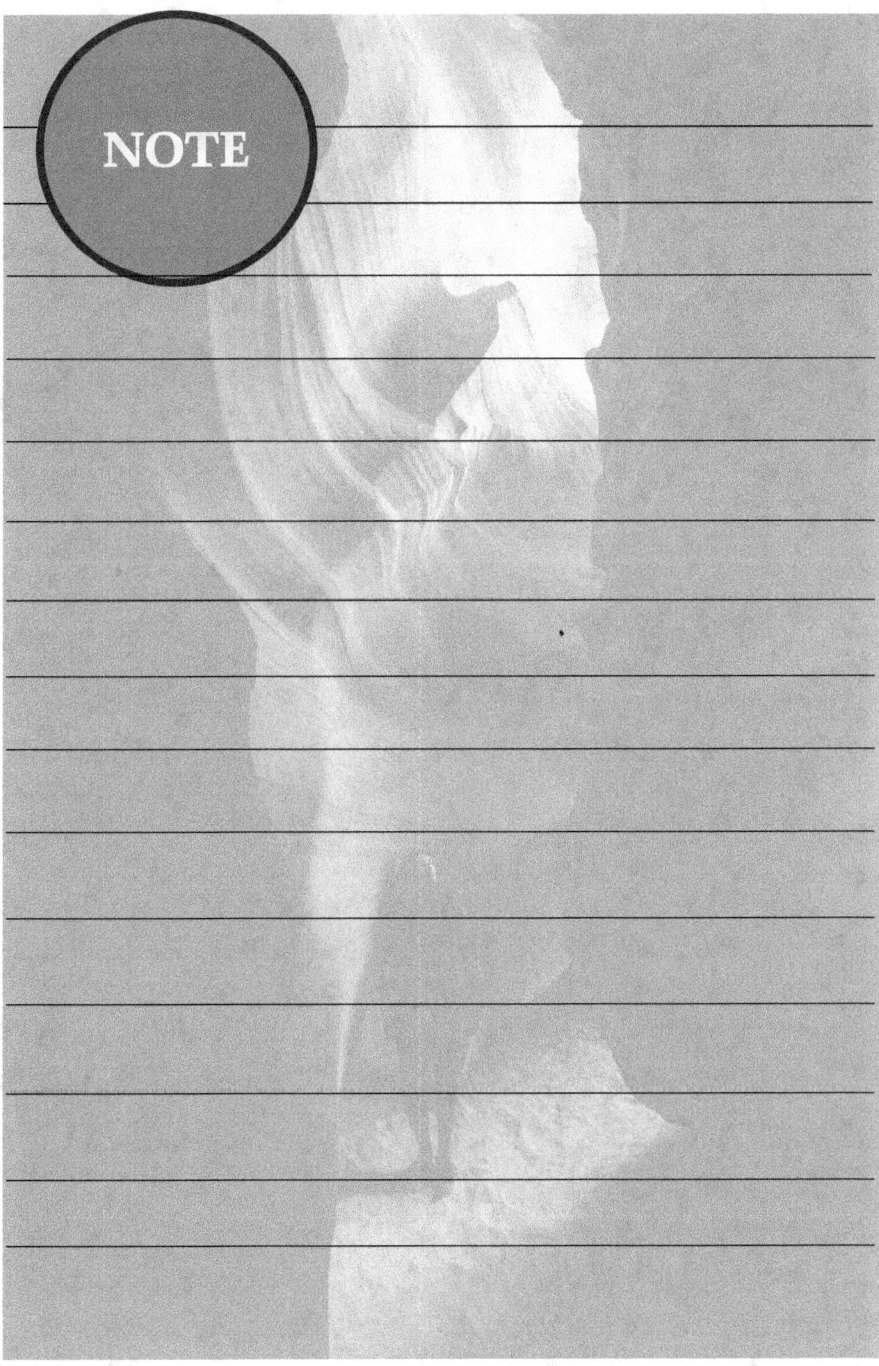
NOTE

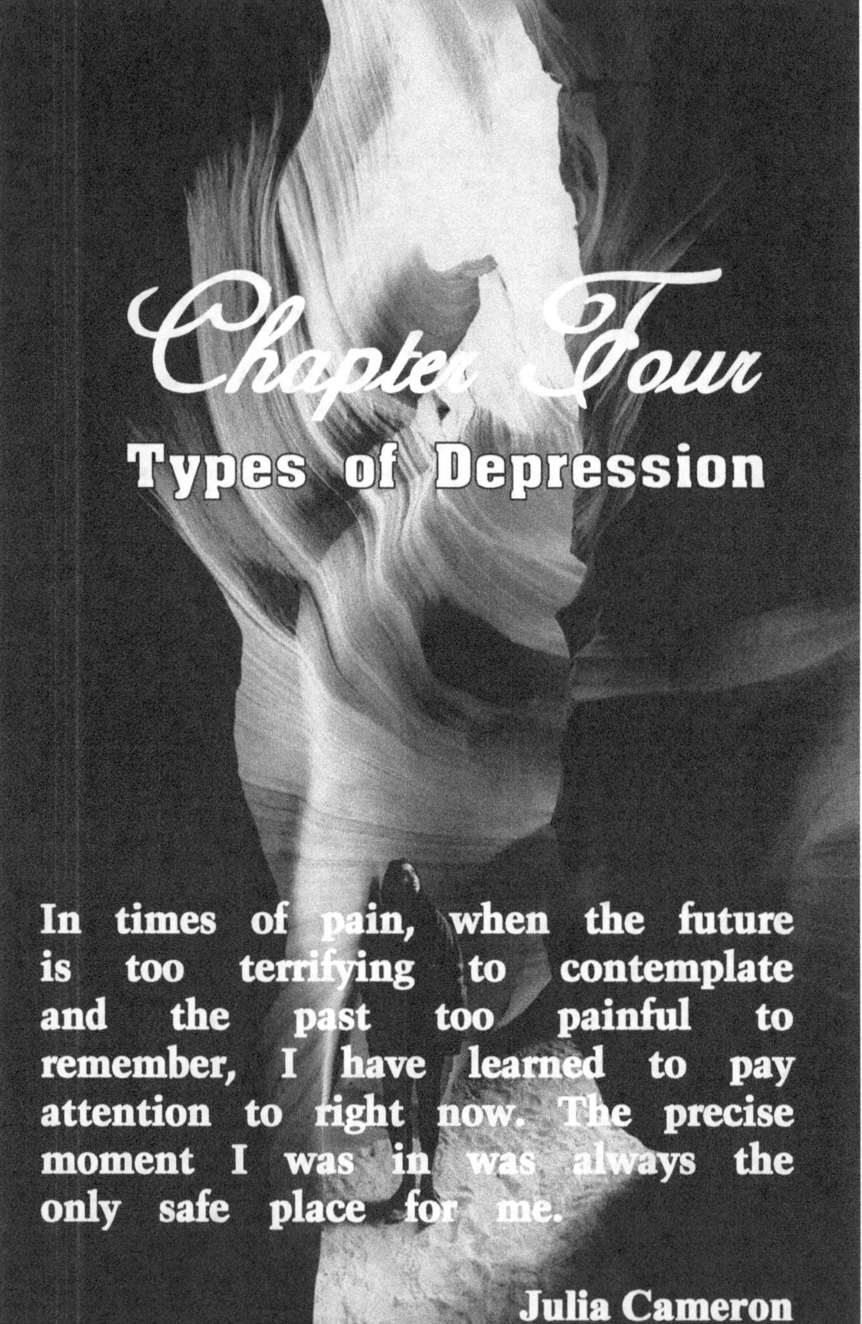
Chapter Four
Types of Depression

In times of pain, when the future is too terrifying to contemplate and the past too painful to remember, I have learned to pay attention to right now. The precise moment I was in was always the only safe place for me.

Julia Cameron

Chapter 4

TYPES OF DEPRESSION

Depression can be described as mood disorders which have physical and mental symptoms. A depressed person lives life as though he/she is living with no reason on earth, then, an idea of ending it all (suicide) feels one's brain. It feels as though everyone around is correct, while the depressed sees nothing good about him/herself. An individual's experience with depression differs based on age. In this section, we look at some types of depression.

Major Depression: Major depression is a serious illness that is characterized by a combination of signs and symptoms that manifest in a toned frame of a minimum of two weeks. Generally, it affects relationships with family members, work or school life and activities, feeding habits, and the person's general health among other symptoms. A major disorder is likened to the harmful effects of diabetes on the human body.

An individually may feel unhappy and be in an irritable mood, inability to work, sleep, eat, and enjoy gratifying activities others do, distress in sleeping habit among other symptoms. Disabling episodes of depression can happen once, twice, or a few times in an individual's lifetime.

A Major Depression Disorder (MDD) is described by scenes of progressively relentless and unavoidable unsettling influences in state of mind. These noticeable changes (above symptoms) happen consistently over two weeks, thus, bringing about overt changes from the individual's past experiences.

After some time, the individual may likewise pull back from social contact and show debilitation in performing normal social jobs. bipolar or unipolar are the major subtypes of MDD.

Bipolar disorder is associated with episodes which change a person's mood, emotion, vitality, action levels, fixation, and the capacity to do everyday activities, which vary from depressive lows to manic highs. Studies are still ongoing to determine the real cause of the bipolar disorder. This illness may be as a result of a combination of some factors which include: genetics, environment and altered brain structure the person's chemistry among other play a role in the illness.

In the past bipolar disorder was called manic-depressive illness or manic depression. Manic episodes may come with these signs and symptoms: high vigour, elated, loss of pleasure in sleeping and rest, loss of touch with the real world activities among others. Depressive episodes may manifest through the following symptoms: low strength, low passion and loss of enthusiasm for everyday exercises. Often, it always comes with a thought to commit suicide. It can stay for some days and even extend to months. Treatment is normally deep-rooted and regularly includes a mix of meds and psychotherapy. Treating this ailment may be a lifelong routine with medications and psychotherapy.

Bipolar disorder is of three types. However, there are conditions other than these three but are still regarded as bipolar disorder. The three types of bipolar disorder have these symptoms which include: clear changes in attitude, vitality, and work levels. These mood swings from times of exceptionally "up," cheerful, bad-tempered, or energetic behaviour (known as a manic episode) to exceptionally "down," tragic, impassive, or sad periods (known as depressive episodes). Less disturbing manic periods are known as hypomanic episodes.

Bipolar I Disorder: it a manic episode that can last for at least 7 days, or by symptoms that are extreme to the point that the individual needs prompt medical care. Generally, depressive episodes happen too it lasts about fourteen days.

Bipolar II Disorder: It is characterized by a form of depressive episodes and hypomanic episodes, yet not the full-blown manic episodes that are common of Bipolar I Disorder.

Cyclothymic Disorder (Cyclothymia): this is characterized by hypomanic symptoms just as times in depressive symptoms which last about two years. It differs in a child as it may be up to one year (in kids and young people). Be that as it may, these symptoms do not meet the prerequisites for hypomanic episodes and depressive episodes respectively.

However, an individual may encounter manifestations of bipolar disorder that don't correlate the three classes recorded above, which is alluded to as "other determined and vague bipolar and related issue."

Unipolar Disorder; this can either be Melancholic or endogenous depression, which is related to explicit clinical signs, especially difficulty in psychomotor capability. Albeit, melancholic sorrow is uncommon in the community, it responds best to thermophysical medicines, for example, antidepressant medications and electroconvulsive and treatment.

Residual depression is another division of unipolar disorder, these, according to Goldberg, are different disorders which include adjustment disorder, depressed mood', 'reactive depression', and to and personality style, or DSM-IV disorder, examples include, dysthymia and cyclothymia.

Dysthymic Disorder: is a less serious type of depression, but more chronic (a long-lasting type of depression when compared to major depression; these do not render a person inoperative but prevent the affected person from functioning optimally, or from feeling good. Sometimes, people with Dysthymia may experience episodes of depressed mood and major depression. The combination of the two is known as 'double-depression." PDD symptoms are the following:

- feelings of displeasure

- Loss of delight in pleasure and interest in activities

- Anger and fretfulness

- Feelings of guilt

- Low self-confidence

- Trouble falling or staying asleep

- Sleeping excessively

- Feelings hopeless

- Fatigue and feeling of being in need

Postpartum depression (PPD): this is depression associated with childbirth and postnatal mood disorder. These covers brief episodes of depressive mood, MDD and baby blues (post-partum) psychosis in which psychotic signs are additionally present.

Pregnancy can realize huge hormonal movements that can regularly influence a woman's mind-sets. Depression can set in at the beginning, during pregnancy or following the birth of a child. Temperament changes, tension, peevishness, and different symptoms are not uncommon during conception effects. These symptoms can last as long as about fourteen days. It is very serious and enduring.

It is very serious and enduring. PPD symptoms include:

- Feeling lacking or useless

- Low temperament, sentiments of pity

- Uneasiness and fits of anxiety

- Extreme changes in mood

- Repulsive to social activities

- Loss of enthusiasm for things you used to appreciate

- Inconvenience holding your child

- Feeling vulnerable and miserable

- Considerations of harming yourself or your child

- Considerations of self-destruction (suicide)

PPD can be dangerous if it is left untreated, the condition can last as long as a year. Medications like antidepressants and hormone treatment can be helpful. PPD can go from a constant dormancy and misery that requires clinical treatment as far as possible up to baby blues psychosis, a condition where the state of mind scene is joined by disarray, mental trips, or dreams.

Premenstrual Dysphoric Disorder: It is a serious and incapacitating type of premenstrual disorder which affect about 1.8–5.8% of women. The disorder is a combination of behavioural, emotional and physical symptoms that repeat monthly during the period of the menstrual cycle of a female. This happens to women from their adolescents stages up till menopause, with an exception during breastfeeding, pregnancy hypothalamic amenorrhea.

Its symptoms include seriously exhausted, Feeling pitiful and miserable; feelings of being under serious stress or tension; changes in emotion, regularly crying and Peevishness; struggling with focusing, among others.

Seasonal Affective Disorder (SAD): is a depressive disorder that is pattern along a particular season or occasionally manifest. A person is experiences depression, and gain weight during the spring season (winter), but during the spring, he/she feels normal. This may not be obtainable everywhere, but in places here;

the condition climatic is mostly cloudy (less on sunlight) at a certain period of the year.

Mourning: It is signs and indications of sadness that happen following the passing of a friend or family member. It is considered as deprivation except if the patients "endure for over two months or incorporate checked utilitarian

disability, sullen distraction with uselessness, self-destructive ideation, maniacal side effects or psychomotor impediment." Emotional clutters or temperament issue are terms that can be utilized to portray every one of those disarranges that is described by the state of mind unsettling influence.

Aggravations can be toward raised extensive enthusiastic state or the other way, i.e., in a discouraged passionate state. Occasional emotional confusion is a subtype of temperament issue where there is a regular example of a state of mind variety. There is a normal example of beginning and abatement of burdensome side effects and scenes, which typically have to begin in fall/ winter and abatement in spring/summer. The side effects of occasional full of a feeling issue are a run of the mill of despondency, frequently including hypersomnia, starch desiring just as expanded hunger and weight gain.

Tension is a disagreeable inclination of dread and worry went with by expanded physiological excitement. Uneasiness issue is those in which dread or then again pressure is the essential aggravation, incorporate phobic issue, alarm scatter, summed up tension issue, over the top issue and post-horrendous stress issue.

Atypical depression: is referred to depression that temporarily goes away in reaction to a momentarily comfortable situation. It is also referred to as major depressive disorder (MDD) with atypical symptoms.

Atypical depression may not be easily noticed in a person, neither by his/herself nor by people around. Atypical depression symptoms include:

- Excessive food consumption and weight gain

- Inordinate feeding sleeping

- Weakness, and feeling "weighed down"

- Intense sensitivity to rejection

- Strong reactive moods etc.

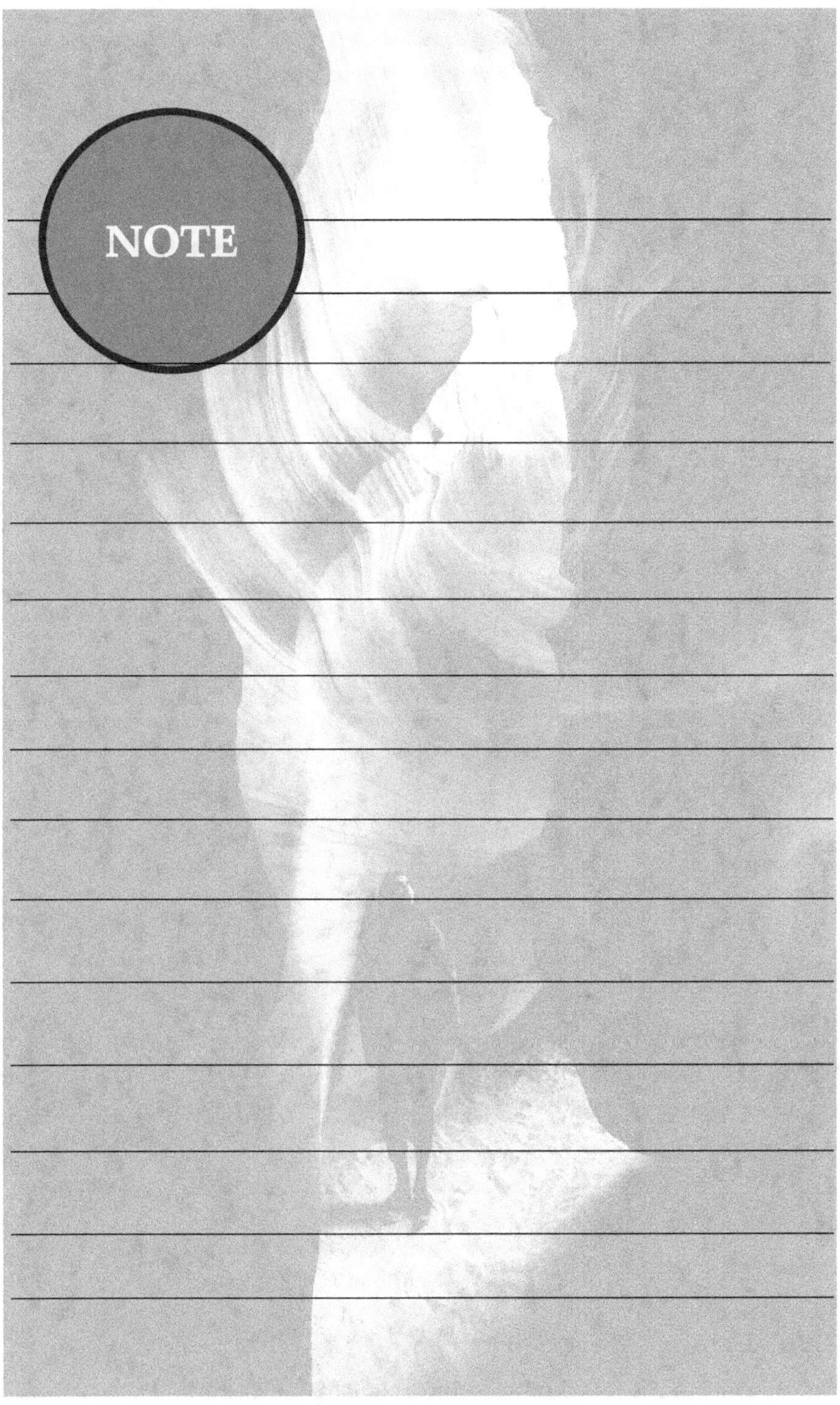

NOTE

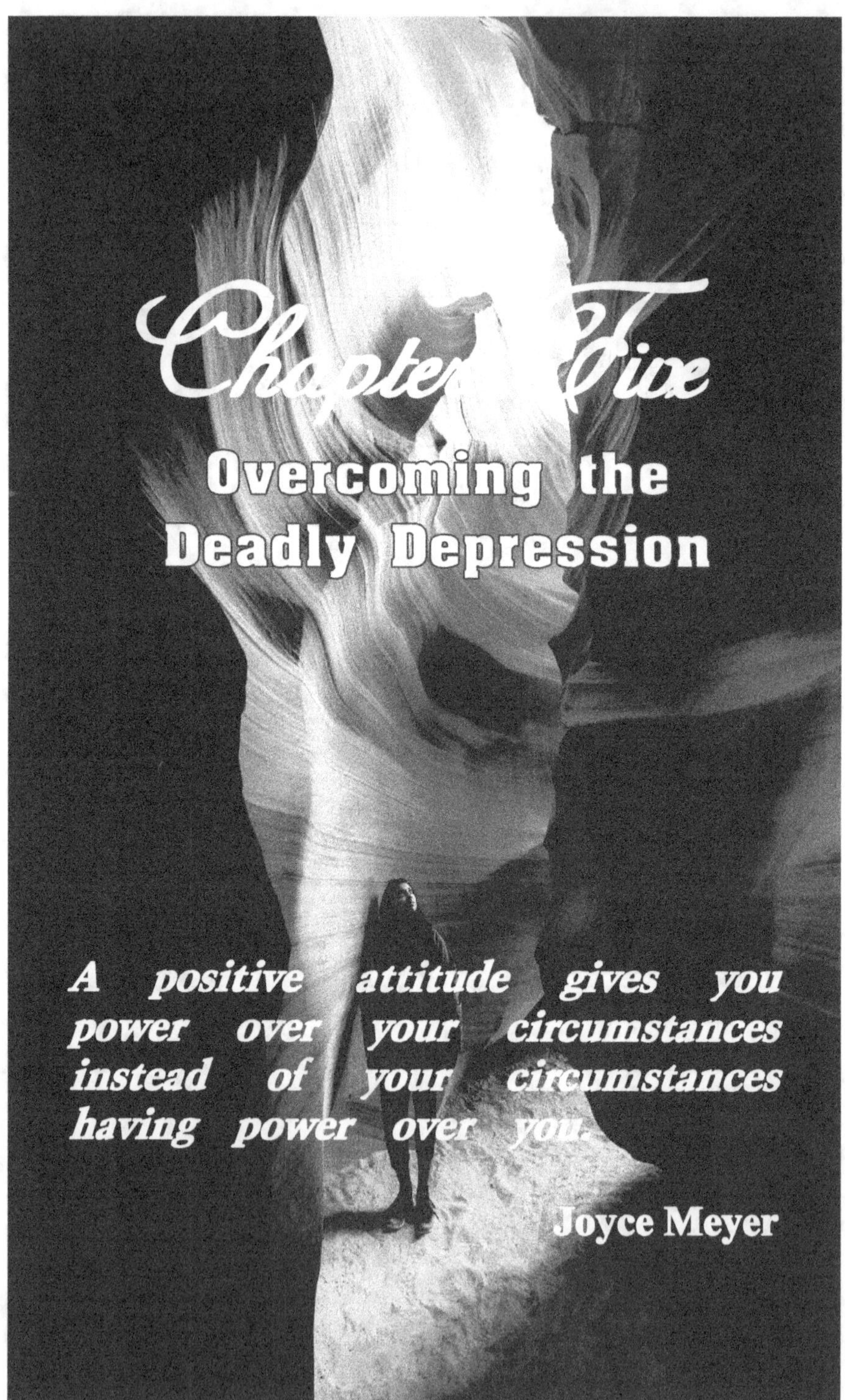
Chapter Five
Overcoming the
Deadly Depression

A positive attitude gives you
power over your circumstances
instead of your circumstances
having power over you.

Joyce Meyer

Chapter 5

OVERCOMING THE DEADLY DEPRESSION

From the above, the whole idea of depression is to steal into a person's mind/brain and take charge. This chapter takes a further look at the most dangerous or deadly depression around which man has to contend with.

Depression is likened to a thief and killer illness whose purpose majorly is to kill or destroy the human mind. The human mind is a focal point or the gateway to depression. Your thoughts then become very critical as it gives access to your minds.

There are many nefarious signs and symptoms of depression as discuss earlier, but among the types, signs and symptoms, which is the most deadly. While we seek better perspectives and answers to this, it is worth to know that a "stitch in time saves nine".

You may have consistently been wondering about the main cause of depression. The real cause of the cause of depression! Sorry, no one is specific as to ascertain the real cause of depression, but it may be as a result of combinations of series of events in our life, most regretful and unforgettable ones. However, continuous difficulties, such as unemployment, loss of a job, being with an uncaring partner or in uncaring relationships, loss of loved ones, loneliness, work stress among other uneventful situations in life, help excrete these bitter memories in our minds. Sometimes, humans are helpless, having pondered on these life challenges, the results are mostly headaches, or end up in tears, having a pillow as a comfort.

However, recent scientific studies in humans' brain have linked the seat of your feelings (emotion) to the brain; stating that certain regions of the mind help the direct state of mind (mood). Nerve cell links, nerve cell development, and the working of nerve circuits majorly affect depression. Howbeit, their thoughts of the neurological underpinnings of disposition (mood) are deficient.

Increasingly sophisticated styles of brain imaging which include positron emission tomography (PET), single-photon emission computed tomography (SPECT), and functional magnetic resonance imaging (fMRI) — help to in no little way to have a closer look at the workings of the human brain. An fMRI examination, for instance, can track changes that take place whilst a region of the brain responds during various tasks. Likewise, a PET or

SPECT test can map the brain by measuring the distribution and density of neurotransmitter receptors in particular areas.

Technology has further helped and given a better insight of which brain region control mood and the way other functions, which includes memory, can be effected through depression. These areas in the brain are most affected and play enormous functions in depression. They are: the amygdala, the thalamus, and the hippocampus

Sometimes, an individual is helpless, and the worries of life keep piling up in the trash. When it started, one may think, 'oh! It is just a loss of a job,' 'it's just a divorce', I think I can cope being alone since nobody appreciates me', thus, winks away at the situation in the name of better days are ahead. But, between now and then, these burdens soon catch up with an individual. And the container/trash keeps increasing. At a point in time, an individual can no longer endure nor cope. The trash can/container is full; no place anymore to absorb the pressure. At this stage, it is extremely overwhelmed. The dirt has been well managed and later struggled with starts littering the environment. It becomes so obvious that that environment is stinky. Same is an application to some who is experiencing depression, you begin to see the effect of what they have been enduring or hiding for a long time.

These causes may be as a result of family history or genetics, low self-worth, serious medical illness (this can cause a serious pain), or alcohol and drug use; in Australia, over 500,000 people experience depression which came as a result of drugs and substances problem.

Previous chapters have discussed the types and symptoms of depression extensively. If I may ask, what is the deadliest depression you can think about (even ones not covered in the book)? Let me help you with some of the lists this book covers; *Atypical depression, Seasonal Affective Disorder (SAD), Premenstrual Dysphoric Disorder, Postpartum depression (PPD), Dysthymic Disorder, Unipolar Disorder, Bipolar disorder, Major Depression.*

Going by the symptoms of these depressions you may want to say one is the deadliest above others, and the argument continues. Let me burst your mind from a pragmatic experience about depression. There is no deadly depression anywhere. The only thing is that failure to address the very small symptoms of depression piles up until it goes out of hand. The next chapter discusses your diagnosis and treatment of depression.

If an individual would nip out the root of depression at an early stage; either in thoughts or life challenges. Stigmatization is another issue of people suffering from depression. This has kept a lot of people from seeking early support or treatment for depression.

The next chapters make practical approaches which cover a wide area of our social lives, including religious solutions to depression and anxiety. Whichever the case, you can be well again.

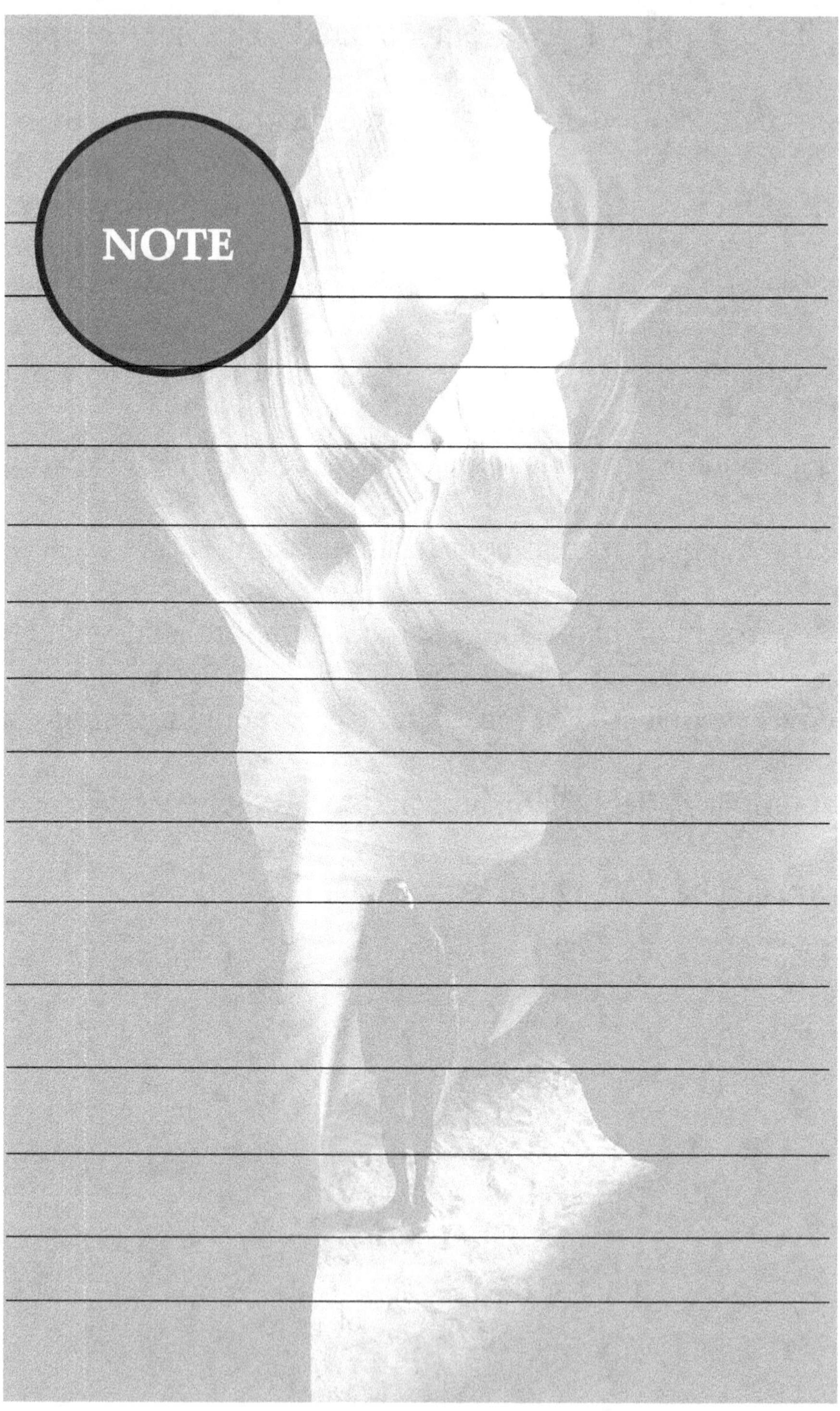
NOTE

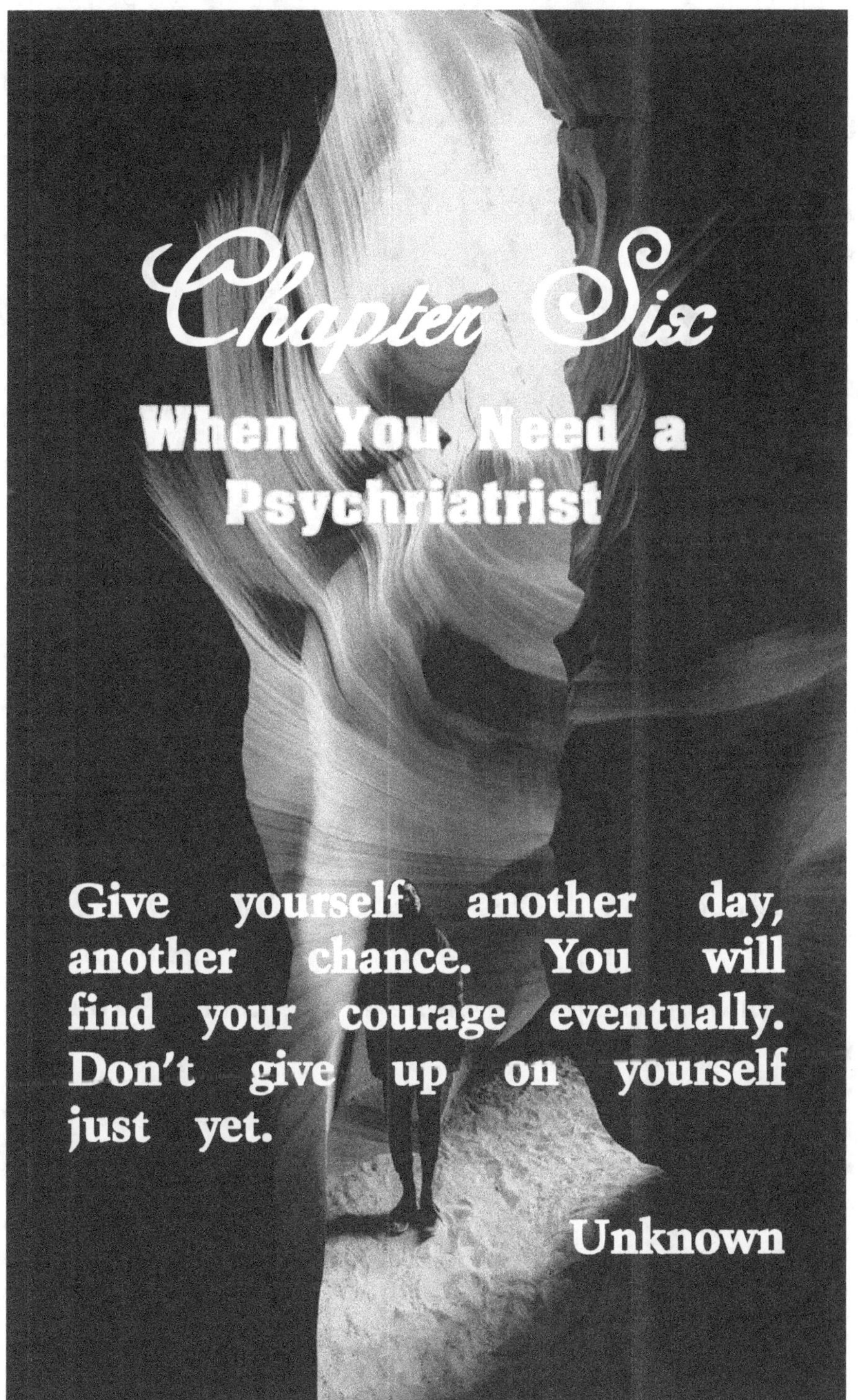
Chapter Six
When You Need a
Psychiatrist

Give yourself another day,
another chance. You will
find your courage eventually.
Don't give up on yourself
just yet.

Unknown

Chapter 6

WHEN YOU NEED A PSYCHRIATRIST

Who do you run to for help when you discovered that you have symptoms of depression? This is a question that can be on itself confusing on what to do and knowing where to begin. Regardless of what the case is, you should be considering consulting a family doctor at an earlier stage. By that, professionals like a doctor or counsellor can be helpful by referring you to a psychiatrist. You can also find out help by joining a like-minded group or health organizations that give support to your health condition, thereby giving you sufficient referrals to best professionals (psychiatrists) who you can communicate your feelings with. Remember that you deserve the right to get the right assistance concerning your health status in relations to depression. Like every normal person, you need to feel loved. But whichever your case is, just know you are not alone.

Your first visit ought to be to your family doctor for an intensive health check. Your family doctor additionally will preclude a few ailments that can cause indications of depression. These could be deficiencies in vitamin and mineral in the body, female hormonal changes, and thyroid conditions. Moreover, a few drug prescriptions may bring about reactions, such as depression in the body. However, If your doctor doesn't discover any of these variables as a reason for your depression, you may then be referred to a psychiatrist, psychologist, or counsellor.

It's significant particularly if this is your first time seeing a medical expert for depression, this, which may come as a referral if your physician suspects depression. Even though your family doctor may offer to prescribe you an antidepressant, does not make him/her the best-qualified specialist to treat depression. She/he can't offer you psychotherapy nor is she knowledgeable about the subtleties of giving prescription on psychotropic drugs.

In the field of Psychiatry, treating depression goes beyond merely giving somebody a prescription on antidepressants and turn them out the door. A few people will require several trials of various prescriptions to discover one that best calms their symptom with minimal measure of side effect. A few people will require more than one medicine to neutralize side effect or to support favourable outcomes; most will likely be beneficial by including psychotherapy.

Talking about these alternatives with your primary care physician will decide the best way.

The role of a mental health professional cannot be overemphasized in dealing with depression, they are is accustomed to seeing experience and diagnosis daily which at the end has given more experience than a family doctor Who may see your symptoms as a puzzle to contend with over some time.

There is a possibility that new patients may want to visit a counsellor or psychologist for their underlying psychological health assessment instead of a psychiatrist. This can be valuable for some individuals, particularly in a situation where the case is still mild. Nonetheless, this is enough, giving reason you should not consider meeting a psychiatrist. A psychiatrist is a medical specialist who can prescribe medication. On the off chance that your depression originates from a chemical irregularity, talk treatment therapy won't be adequate to treat you. At this point, you should consider visiting a psychiatrist, who can both prescribe drugs and offer you psychotherapy if it is required. These two approaches to the prescription of medicine and talk therapy are most valuable to patients.

Who is a psychiatrist?

A psychiatrist is a clinical specialist (medical doctor) who is an authority (specialist) in mental and psychological waitress. He/she has expertise in diagnosing and treating individuals with mental sickness. Psychiatrists have a profound knowledge of physical and psychological well-being; and how they affect another. They help individuals with emotional health conditions which include: addiction, schizophrenia, depression, bipolar disorder, dietary problems among others.

There are many explanation individuals search for psychiatrists. They seek them for issues that bother on; difficulties in adjusting after significant life changes or stress which affect them; nervousness, fear or stress; continuous feeling of depression and low mood; self-destructive thoughts (suicide); thoughts of harming; harming yourself intentionally; an excessive amount of vitality, being not able to rest, wind down or calm down; obsessed with negative thoughts; having an inclination that individuals are after you or need to hurt you; violence, disturbance or emotional upheavals; insomnia; poor focus and concentration, hyperactivity; issue betting, gaming or other addictive practices; issues around self-image, and of eating well; memory crisis; wild a or medication use; having any worrisome problem in your relationship, spouse, lover, or others; mental trips (hearing or seeing things that aren't there) and other sleeplessness issues, these among other reasons.

It is worthy to note that, in a situation, you have come to the level of being overwhelmed with depression and can no longer deal with anymore, you will need to look for some professional assistance from a veteran psychiatrist. Other related professionals like counsellors, psychologist or your spiritual adviser may also be helpful. In a situation you are indisposed to looking for this kind of help, you ought to have a good friend who you can request to go with you to the doctor or a psychiatrist. Peradventure you don't have any friend; you can look for help from religious leaders you know or primary health care centre. There are many care groups out there that can get you out with certain issues in particular. The groups are free, when you join, we will see people who have similar issues with you and rob minds together.

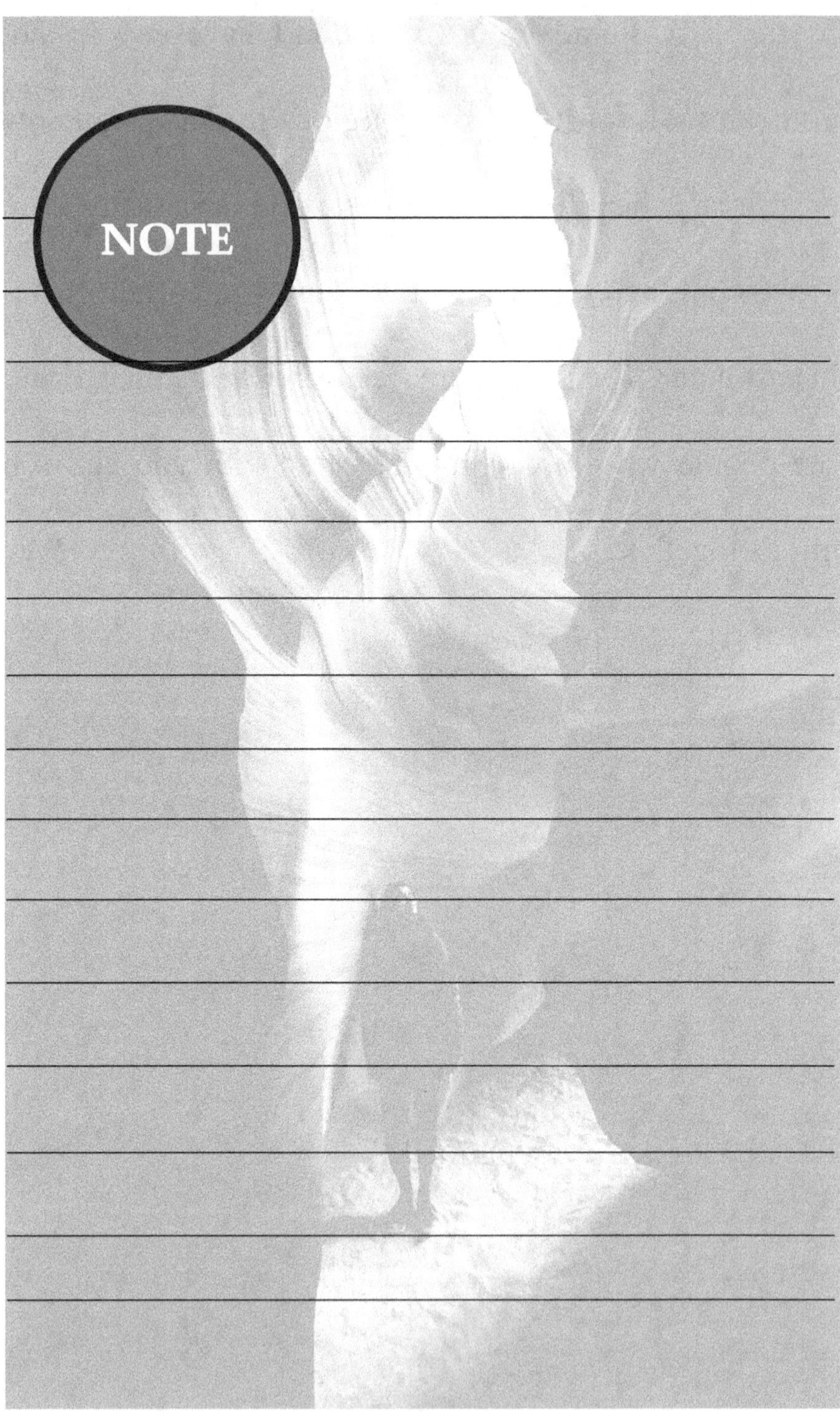

NOTE

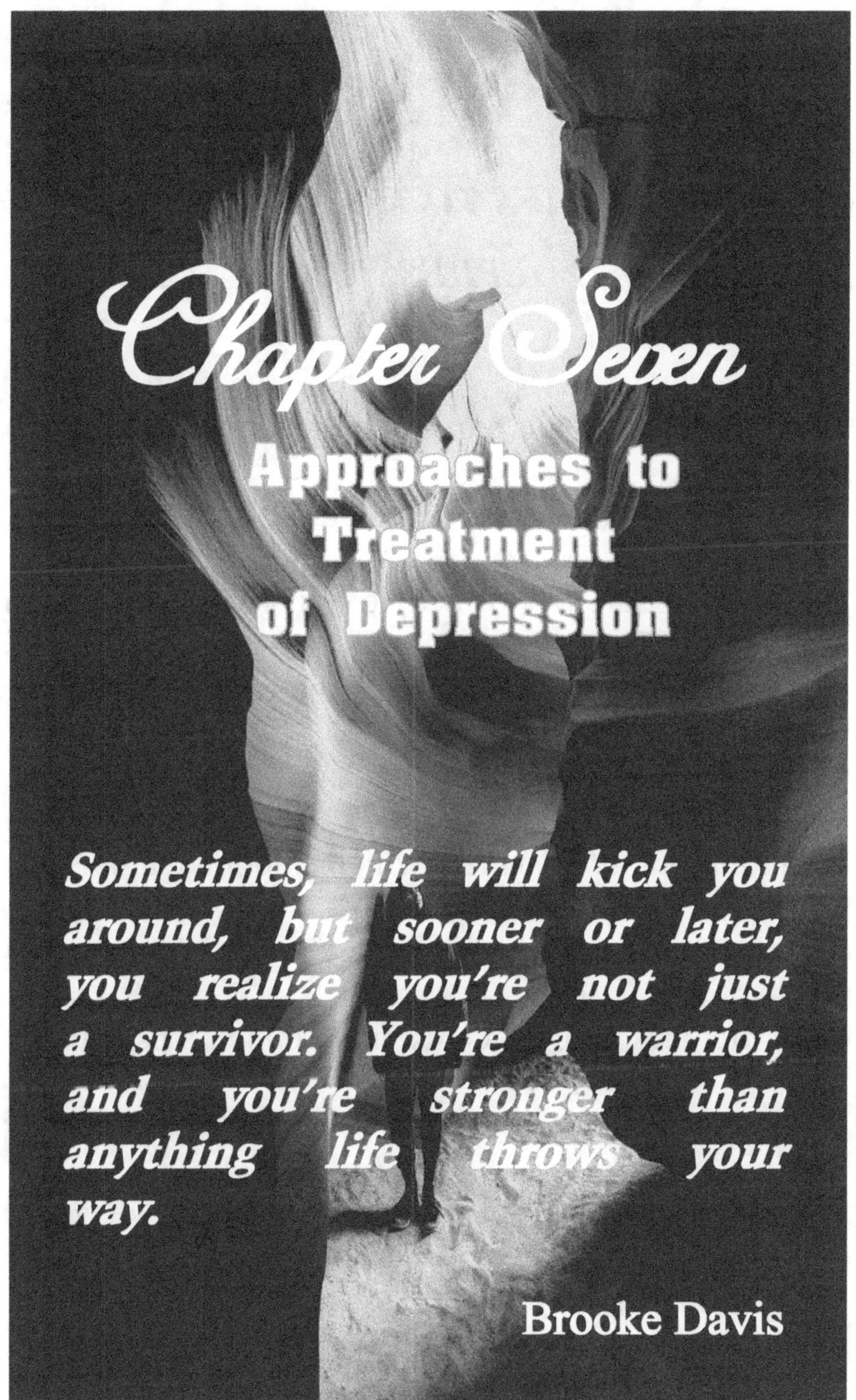
Chapter Seven

Approaches to
Treatment
of Depression

Sometimes, life will kick you
around, but sooner or later,
you realize you're not just
a survivor. You're a warrior,
and you're stronger than
anything life throws your
way.

Brooke Davis

Chapter 7

APPROACHES TO TREATMENT OF DEPRESSION

Depression is a treatable sickness, but many do not know this. Research has shown that only about 10% of people living with depression seek a solution to this illness. Some of the reasons for this may be stimulation, enduring the depressive symptoms or circumstances with the notion that it is just one of those issues one have to live with for the rest of one's life, lack of confidence in a country's psychiatric hospital and poor government policies to adequately care for patients, inability to make appropriate diagnose and give successful treatment to patients.

Many who do not perceive depression as a serious illness, this mild illness at the initial stage can be devastating, which, whenever left unchecked, it may prompt other clinical illnesses. MDD specifically is related to several several interminable physical ailments, including joint inflammation (arthritis), cardiovascular disease, diabetes, chronic respiratory disease, hypertension, cancer, asthma, and various chronic pain conditions.

Considering the above, it is imperative to give extraordinary consideration to diagnose and treat depression among individuals with the underlying health condition to save the lives of such patients. Thoughts of committing suicide seem to be the best solution because of unimaginable pains go through.

For the treatment of most patients with major depression, a blend of pharmacotherapy and psychotherapy is viewed as a compelling way to deal with the treatment. The decision to use antidepressant in clinical treatment depends on the idea of neurobiological factors liable for depression. In this way, antidepressant drugs are intended to affect distinctive neurotransmitter frameworks of the brain. These biological frameworks incorporate serotonin, norepinephrine, dopamine, and different kinds of neurotransmitters related indications, a right dosage will be prescribed to control an inefficiency in the neurotransmitter frameworks and improve the condition of depression.

The decision of antidepressant for treatment relies upon the kind of depression that a patient experiences. The choice of antidepressant prescription varies because of the different types of depression patients are faced with.

Before antidepressant drugs can be prescribed, variable factors of depression are put into consideration and the side effect of the drugs in the light of the peculiarity of the type of patient depression. A few patients may require a mix of antidepressants, contingent upon the seriousness of the sickness and its protection from treatment. At the point when a patient experiences despondency with maniacal symptoms, an antipsychotic medication might be required.

For a depression triggered by a family or social incidence, psychotherapy and a critical thinking approach may be satisfactory except if the force of depression or different reasons direct that various measures be taken.

Biological Approach

The Biological Approach to dealing with psychopathology agrees that mental has a biological or physical cause. The focal approach is based on hereditary/genetic qualities, neurophysiology, neurotransmitters, neuroanatomy among others. Any type of treatment for the mental disturbance that endeavours to modify physiological operation, including drug dosage/treatment, electroconvulsive treatment (psychosurgery).

This approach contends that psychological disorder is identified with the physical structure and mind workings. Conditions such as hallucinations, suicide thoughts or outrageous feelings of fear among other symptoms can be distinguished as mental illness. These health conditions put together brought about the ailment in the body. These symptoms help the specialist to determine if a patient is experiencing an extreme psychosis.

Schizophrenia is an illness that is related to severe psychosis. It can be genetic/hereditary, biochemistry, Neuroanatomy, or Neuroendocrine factors.

Psychotherapy/Psychological treatments for depression

Psychological treatment (psychotherapy) is another approach to treating depression. It can assist you with changing your reasoning pattern and improve your adapting aptitudes so you're better positioned to manage life's anxieties, stresses and conflicts. Psychotherapy can likewise assist you with remaining great by recognizing and changing awkward thoughts and conducts.

There are a number of compelling psychotherapy treatment for depression, also various delivery choices. A few people may want to work one on one with an expert, while others get progressively out during a group gathering session.

Cognitive Behaviour Therapy (CBT)

Cognitive behaviour therapy is an organized mental treatment which known to be one of the best and most known treatments normally used treatment for depression. It is a treatment that has to do with cognition and conduct; an attitudinal change in reasoning, thoughts and actions toward positive gains and improved feelings. It has been seen as valuable for a wide period of time, including kids, young people, grown-ups and older people.

A medical advisor assists you with recognizing the negative thoughts domicile in you. Thoughts such as: 'I am useless', 'I can't do anything right', 'I'll never feel much improved', 'this circumstance will never improve' among other negative thoughts, can be changed with progressively reasonable thoughts that help your well-being and life goals. CBT ordinarily doesn't concentrate on the past, however on changing your thoughts, emotions, and practices at the moment.

The hallmark of this approach is to help you build responses that are increasingly reasonable, positive, critical thinking and a positive mindset. It can also be done electronically (c-treatments).

Interpersonal therapy (IPT)

IPT is organized psychotherapy that centres on issues relating to personal relationships and the skills to manage such. IPT depends on the possibility that relationship issues can add to the cause of depression, sometimes, even the cause; it can as well significantly affect someone having depression.

IPT can help you perceive or recognize patterns in your personal and social relationships which make you continually powerless against depression. Recognizing these patterns implies you can concentrate on improving relationships, managing despondency and finding better approaches to coexist with others.

IPT claimed that suitable, stable social help is very important to an individual's general welfare. As a result, when a person vacillates, an individual usually experiences the negative and awfulness of that relationship. Thus, this therapy tries to improve an individual's relationship skills, for example, a successful skill, communicating feelings/emotions properly, and being aptly emphatic in personal and professional circumstances. The administration of IPT is similar to CBT which can be done with an individual or in a group setting.

Behaviour therapy/ Behavioral activation therapy (BA)

Unlike CBT, BA, does not endeavour to change beliefs or one's perceptions, rather, it centres on developing and encouraging excrcises or activities that are keened to one's interest; satisfying, or rewarding, as such bringing about withdrawal from patterns that do not interest a person. Thus, versing negative patterns like avoidance, lethargy and inactivity that make depression worse.

these exercises could be spending your time with friends and family or taking a yoga class. BA is a practical approach that helps you distinguish your goals, and accomplish them. BA may also be successful in a gathering group.

Problem-solving therapy (PST)

PST helps people with sadness figure out how to adapt adequately to upsetting issues in everyday lives. Individuals with depression may see problems as dangers and accept that they are unable to overcome them. A therapist will assist with defining the issue, conceptualize elective sensible solutions, select supportive solutions, and objectively implement and assess it.

Family or Couples Treatment

Family or Couples Treatment can be a choice when depression is directly influencing family structures or members or the well-being of important relationships. This therapy centres on the interpersonal connections among relatives/family and looks to guarantee that the mode of communication model adopted is clear to everyone involved. Additionally analyzed the roles of different members of a family play in strengthening your depression. Furthermore, everybody is given basic training for depression.

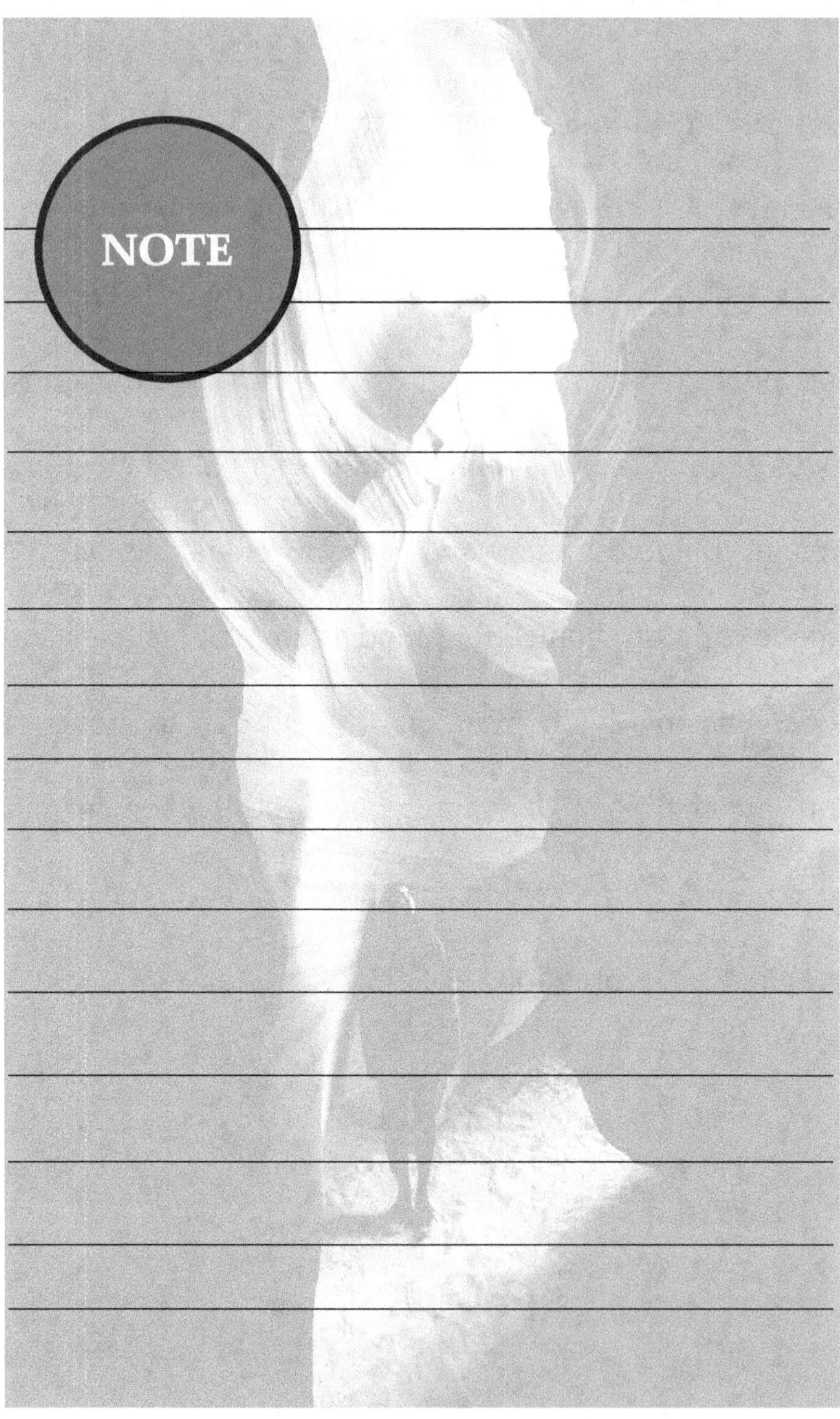
NOTE

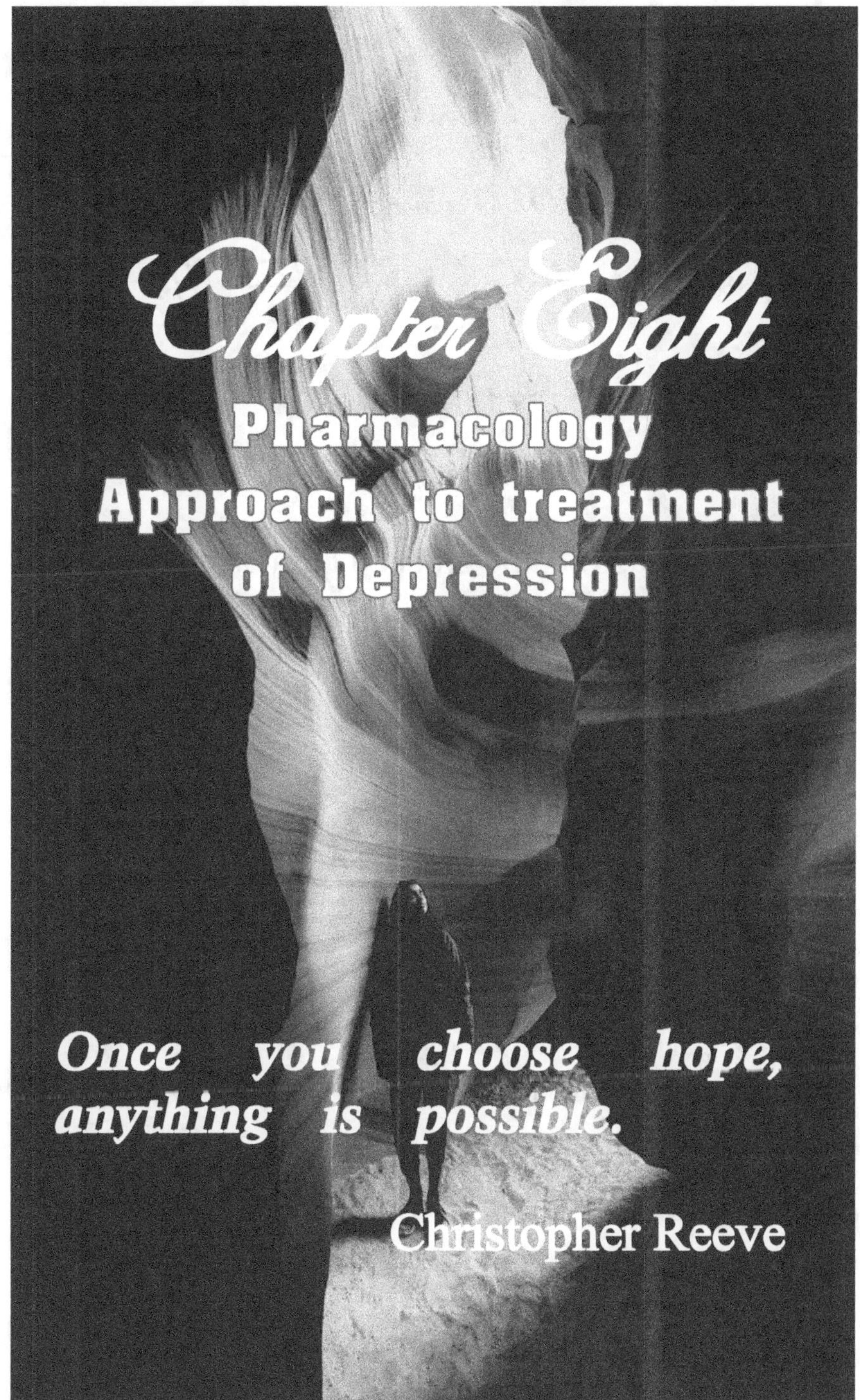
Chapter Eight
Pharmacology
Approach to treatment
of Depression
Once you choose hope,
anything is possible.
Christopher Reeve

Chapter 8

PHARMACOLOGY APPROACH TO TREATMENT OF DEPRESSION

The treatment of depression depends on the usage of drugs drawn from various classes. Drugs can be grouped by their structure (for example, tricyclic antidepressants (TCAs) or their component of action (for example, monoamine reuptake restraint versus monoamine oxidase inhibition). Most medications as of now endorsed follow up on monoaminergic transmission. The beginning of clinical potency is for the least period of 2–3 weeks after commencement of treatment for all antidepressant prescriptions. This demonstrates that it is not the quick changes that follow the acute administration of these mixtures that are liable for their remedial effects but delay in the secondary effects.

Here are some of the drugs used for the treatment of depression are the following:

- Selective serotonin reuptake inhibitors (SSRIs)

- Serotonin/norepinephrine reuptake inhibitors (SNRIs)

- Atypical antidepressants

- Tricyclic antidepressants (TCAs)

- Serotonin-Dopamine Activity Modulators (SDAMs)

- N-methyl-D-aspartate (NMDA)

- Monoamine oxidase inhibitors (MAOIs)

Selective Serotonin Reuptake Inhibitors (SSRIs)

Selective serotonin reuptake inhibitors are a broadly used kind of antidepressant. They are the most prescribed for the treatment of depression. Especially in severe or persistent cases, and are regularly used with psychotherapy like cognitive behavioural therapy (CBT).

SSRIs are normally the principal choice drug for depression since they have fewer side effects than most different kinds of antidepressant. Basic side impacts of SSRIs are gastrointestinal upset, sexual dysfunctions, and changes in vitality level (i.e. tiredness, worries).

The SSRIs are believed to be moderately unproblematic in patients with cardiovascular sickness, as these do not seem to affect blood pressure, pulse (heart rate), cardiac conduction, or heartbeat. Be that as it may, time-dependent QT prolongation has been accounted for with citalopram.

Although some government agencies in charge of food and drugs, like in the US, do not recommend the use of citalopram for patients with congenital long QT conditions, nonetheless, citalopram ought to be stopped in patients who are found to have a persistent corrected QT interval (QTc) more than 500 ms.

The use of citalopram ought not to surpass 40 mg/day, given the danger of conceivably deadly cardiovascular arrhythmias; moreover, higher dosages have not been proven to be more potent in treating depression, older patients above years should only take 20 mg/day.

There is a belief that SSRIs work by expanding serotonin levels in the brain. Serotonin could be a connection transmitter (neurotransmitter; a chemical carrier that conveys signals between nerve cells within the cerebrum (brain). It is conceived to impact mood, feelings and rest.

When conveying a message, 5-hydroxytryptamine (serotonin) is often reabsorbed by the nerve cells; "reuptake". SSRIs work by interference ("inhibiting") reuptake, which suggests that a lot of serotonin is accessible to pass additional messages between available nerve cells.

Based on the above, one may not be wrong to say that depression and mental health conditions are caused by low 5-hydroxytryptamine levels, but, increase in the serotonin will improve symptoms and make individuals more receptive to any types of treatment, including CBT. SSRIs include citalopram (Celexa), Fluoxetine (Prozac), Fluvoxamine (Luvox), Paroxetine (Paxil),

Sertraline (Zoloft), Vortioxetine (Brintellix), Escitalopram (Lexapro), Vilazodone (Viibryd).

Serotonin/Norepinephrine Reuptake Inhibitors (SNRIs)

SNRIs can be used as first-line agents, notably in patients with serious weariness or pain syndromes related to the episode of depression. SNRIs even have a significant role. It also works as second-line agents in patients who haven't effectively responded to SSRIs.

However, the combination of SNRIs with other antidepressants could be additional problematic and trigger a negative response.

SNRIs are generally effective for the treatment of depression. They may be an efficient kind of treatment for individuals who have had unsuccessful treatment with SSRIs. SSRIs solely work on one chemical traveller, serotonin. SNRIs may also be a good prescription for individuals with anxiety.

Women who are pregnant or breastfeeding ought to avoid taking SNRIs unless the advantages of taking them outweigh the risks to the mother and baby. Babies delivered to mothers who take SNRIs throughout the second trimester of pregnancy could experience withdrawal symptoms, such as difficult respiratory, feeding issues and tremors. Additionally, SNRIs also passes into breast milk.

While all antidepressants could cause a risk to a developing foetus, definite choices are also safer for a mother and baby. However, you speak with your doctor regarding the most effective choice for you.

Individuals with liver problems or hypertension (blood pressure) may likewise need to avoid SNRIs. These medications can increase blood pressure levels.

On the off chance that you have a liver problem, a greater amount of the drugs may remain in your system longer and lead to an increased danger of side effects.

In a case where you must use it, kindly seek your doctor's advice. Some downsides of SNRIs include queasiness, changes in hunger, muscle weakness, fomentation, heart palpitations, tremor, increased blood pressure, increased pulse (heart rate), migraine, trouble peeing, sleeping disorder, drowsiness, dry mouth, unnecessary sweating, constipation etc.

Some downsides of SNRIs include: nausea, changes in appetite, muscle weakness, tremor, agitation, heart palpitations, difficulty urinating, increased heart rate, headache, increased blood pressure, dizziness, insomnia, sleepiness, dry mouth, excessive sweating, constipation, fluid retention, especially in older adults, an inability to maintain an erection or have an orgasm (in men).

SNRIs drugs include duloxetine (Cymbalta, Irenka), venlafaxine (Effexor), desvenlafaxine (Pristiq), venlafaxine (Effexor XR), duloxetine (Cymbalta), levomilnacipran (Fetzima), atomoxetine (Strattera), milnacipran (Savella), tramadol (Ultram, desvenlafaxine (Pristiq, Khedezla), levomilnacipran (Fetzima).

Atypical antidepressants (TCAs)

Atypical antidepressants are not normal, they don't fit into the same classes of antidepressants. They are exceptional prescriptions that work in various manners from each other.

Atypical antidepressants lessen the effects of depression by inciting chemical transporters (neurotransmitters) used to move signals between the brain cells. Like most antidepressants, atypical antidepressants work by eventually affecting changes in brain component and transmission in brain nerve cell circuit board known to control the mood of an individual; to help reduce depression.

Atypical antidepressants change the intensities of at least one of the neurotransmitters which are; dopamine, serotonin or norepinephrine.

They, however, show low toxicity in overdose.

Bupropion has a bit of advantage over the SSRIs of causing less sexual dysfunctions and less GI trouble.

Mirtazapine is related to the high vulnerability of weight gain, so patients who are treated with this drug should be cautious observing of their weight.

While patients may react to antidepressants, atypical antidepressants are not excluded, however, some people may not encounter any. Some symptoms may leave after a period, while others may lead you and your primary care physician to attempt alternate medicines.

A vast majority of the atypical antidepressants have the following as side effects. These include; dry mouth, dizziness or unsteadiness. A few antidepressants may assist you with sleeping and are best taken in the evening time, while others may deprive you of sleep. Some may cause increased appetite, causing weight gain, while others may cause constipation and sexual dysfunctions. In all, always conduct your doctor.

Some endorsed atypical antidepressants drugs by Food and Medication Organization (FDA) for treating depression include Vortioxetine (Trintellix), Bupropion (Wellbutrin SR, Wellbutrin XL, others), Mirtazapine (Remeron), Nefazodone, Trazodone etc.

Serotonin-Dopamine Activity Modulators (SDAMs)

Aripiprazole (Abilify) and Brexpiprazole (Rexulti) are SDAMs.

Brexpiprazole is known as an adjunctive treatment for major depression disorder (MDD). Aripiprazole is known for schizophrenia, serious treatment of manic and mixed episodes related with bipolar I and serves as an adjunct to MDD, touchiness related to autistic disorder, and treatment of Tourette issue. Additionally, aripiprazole injection acts fast for agitation related to schizophrenia or bipolar mania.

In clinical preliminaries, brexpiprazole has been added to existing antidepressant treatment in patients who had low responses towards various forms of antidepressant treatments. Brexpiprazole (2 mg and 3 mg every day) in addition to antidepressant therapy was better off placebo plus antidepressant therapy on the first stage.

Tricyclic Antidepressants

TCAs were one of the main antidepressants, they are, despite the emergence of other antidepressants very effective in treating depression. These medications are a good choice for individuals whose depression repel the effects of other drugs. Even though cyclic antidepressants can be very effective, some people have attested to their side effects. That is the reason these drugs are not frequently used as a first treatment.

They have a long record of potency in treating depression. They are less used generally considering their side effects profile and their toxicity can be in overdose.

Generally, tricyclic antidepressants are prescribed by clinicians after other drugs proved abortive and could not alleviate the depression condition. Tricyclic antidepressants help keep more serotonin and norepinephrine open to the brain. These chemicals are made normally by your body and are thought to influence your mood. Keeping a greater amount of them accessible to your brain, tricyclic antidepressants help raise your mood. Some tricyclic antidepressants are used to treat different conditions.

Tricyclic antidepressants may cause addition in weight, sedation and constipation uniquely different from other antidepressants. Albeit, various drugs have various effects. If you have inconvenient reactions on one tricyclic antidepressant, tell your physician. Changing to another cyclic antidepressant may help.

Individuals who drink alcohol habitually ought to keep away from tricyclic antidepressants. Liquor reduces the antidepressants reactions of these drugs. It can also bring about an increase in drowsy effects.

TCAs include the following: Amitriptyline (Elavil), Clomipramine (Anafranil), Desipramine (Norpramin), Doxepin (Sinequan), Imipramine (Tofranil), Nortriptyline (Pamelor), Protriptyline (Vivactil), Trimipramine (Surmontil)

Monoamine Oxidase Inhibitors (MAOIs)

MAOIs are a class of prescription used to treat depression. They are one of the first set of primary drugs for depression. But, they're less known these days compared to other despondency drugs, however, some people still prefer using it.

These are generally efficient in a wide scope of affective and anxiety treatment. Because of the danger of hypertensive emergency, patients with prescriptions must follow a low-tyramine diet. Other unfavourable effects include anxiety, insomnia, orthostasis, an increase of weight, and sexual dysfunctions. MAOIs include the following; isocarboxazid (Marplan), phenelzine (Nardil), selegiline (Emsam), and tranylcypromine (Parnate).

Given their side effects which is more than other antidepressants, MAOIs is often the last drug prescribed to patients to treat depression. Some side effects of MAOIs include fatigue, muscle aches, nervousness, insomnia, reduced libido, erectile dysfunction (ED), dizziness, lightheadedness, diarrhoea, dry mouth, high blood pressure, tingling of the skin, difficulty urinating, weight gain.

N-methyl-D-aspartate antagonist

NMDA receptor antagonist esketamine intranasal (Spravato) is a recommended brand of drugs by the FDA as very effective in the treatment of depression. It comes as a nasal spray that is taken under a doctor or pharmacist's supervision (to guide against abuse) with other oral antidepressants.

Spravato is used to treat depression known as treatment-resistant depression (TRD). TRD is a kind of depression that have shown resistance to two or more antidepressant drugs in individuals. It contains the drug, esketamine which is approved only for use in adults with at least one other antidepressant drug that is taken by mouth.

The side effect of Spravato can be mild or grave. Some common side effects of Spravato include Anxiety, dissociation (feeling "out of body"), faintness, feeling drunk, increased blood pressure, fatigue, (extreme tiredness), nausea, unresponsiveness in your hands and feet, sedation (sleepiness, trouble thinking clearly, inability to drive or use heavy machinery), vertigo (feeling like you're moving when you're not), vomiting etc. You can talk to your doctor or pharmacist if you are not with any of the side effects you are experiencing.

NOTE

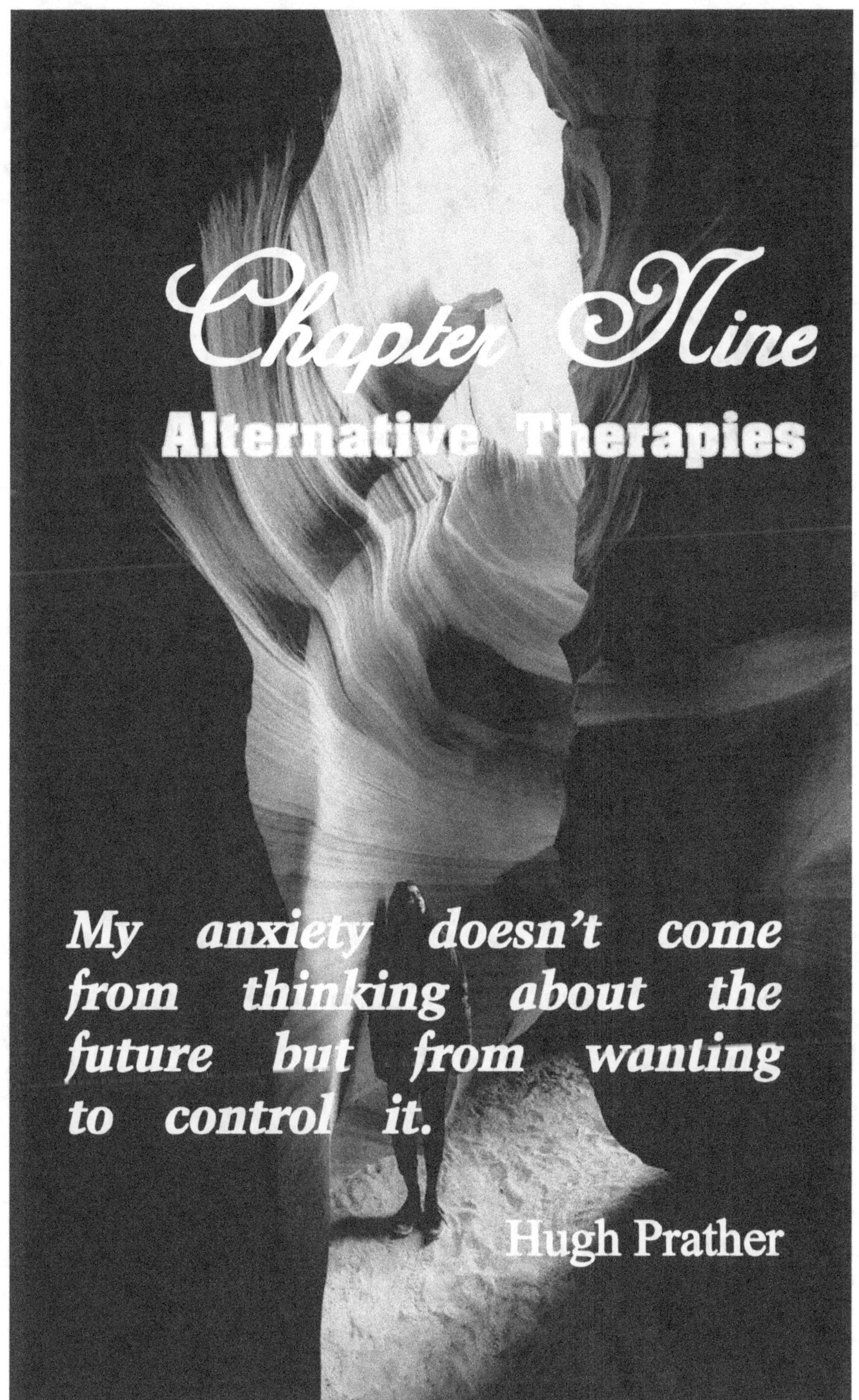
Chapter Nine
Alternative Therapies
My anxiety doesn't come from thinking about the future but from wanting to control it.
Hugh Prather

Chapter 9

ALTERNATIVE THERAPIES

Alternative therapy for depression is a treatment that covers various discipline. It involves the collaborative use of nature, diet, relaxation, massage, yoga herbal remedies, exercise, acupuncture etc. to treat mental conditions and lifestyle. Considering the side effects of some of the scientifically proven effective antidepressants, today, some people may be willing to make use of alternative treatment for depression. There are lots of alternative or herbal drugs out there for treating depression anxiety and other mental health conditions. Some of them are in clinical trials while some have been considered very effective for treating depression and other health conditions, e.g. St. John's Wort etc.

Studies have shown that alternative therapy has soothing effects on the body and mind. Some have considered the effects of alternative therapy as an organic cure for treating depression and anxiety among other mental health issues because when use they directly fit into an individual's nervous system.

While antidepressants can have negative effects on the body and can be highly addictive, one should be very careful in the choice of alternative treatment.

Acupuncture (needle therapy): It's an old Chinese practice in which there are insertions of needles of different lengths into the skin at a particular point in the body. These points are straightly connected to the area of the body that requires treatment. This kind of treatment needs time before some can determine its efficacy.

Massage therapy: it is a therapy that helps to manipulate your muscles by way of softening the tissues to perform optimally and promote relaxation. It is useful and as profoundly powerful in treating depression. Massage therapy can help to relieve tension in your muscles and connective tissues by way of reducing the stiffness or pain in the body muscle area. It can as well help in increasing blood flow and relaxation in the body. Although massage may not in itself alleviate depression, physical symptoms of depression are reduced. Massage helps to reduce back pain, sluggishness, muscle aches, joint pains etc. and helps to reduce fatigue but improve the sleeping problem in an individual.

There are different types of massage; Chair massage (individuals are made to sit and lean forward towards a headrest. It is usually done without clothes removal), Swedish massage (therapists apply smooth, circular, kneading action to the muscles), Deep tissue massage (this focuses on tight muscles which are closer to a person's bones and connective tissues where stress is dominant, Shiatsu massage (this is applied at various body points of needle therapy, i.e. acupuncture), the Neuromuscular massage (this helps in massaging muscles which impact the nervous system). Reflexology (this therapy asserts pressures on muscles in the feet area which connected with other organs of the body. **Aromatherapy** (this is done with scented oil, it boost energy and reduce stress), hot stone (this therapy places stones on the body to relax muscle nerves. Force is often applied in order to reduce stress).

Bright Light Therapy: This is one of the most widely recognized types of alternative treatments, in that when people are exposed to morning sunlight, it can help to generate some natural chemical inside the body. This light works by striking the retina. It initiates a special piece of your brain which is known as the "hypothalamus". The reality is that this part can contrarily affect the sleep cycle and the craving for food in an individual. Also, it can change moods and sex drive. The mix of activities exercise with this treatment can give extraordinary outcomes. On the off chance that you don't get immediate daylight, consider using a lightbox. The SAD or seasonal affective disorder is a sort of depression happening as a result of the nonattendance of sun expose during winter.

In the case of the above condition, Bright Light Therapy can be considered as the most appropriate. There are various kinds of herbal supplements that you can try for your treatment. Must be careful, put in perspective the state of your liver. They must be of good quality.

Vitamins (D): vitamins are very useful in reducing stress. They can be obtained from natural products, vegetables and supplements. Vitamin B has been proven to be very efficient in mind and soul related health conditions. You can consider using magnesium, zinc or folic acid for effectively managing your stress-related depression issues. While are also herbs are also good, they may hurt certain kinds of drugs. Yet, ensure that they meet the most basic pharmaceutical standards.

However, research has proven that Vitamin D helps in reducing the chance of having depression in children. Exposing a child to adequate sunlight and consumption of meals rich in Vitamin B help to reduce the risk of a child from suffering from depression later in life. Researchers believe that children with a low level of Vitamin D are susceptible to suffering from a mental health problem, such as depression when they are teenagers. The study stated that children who had enough Vitamin D showed a ten per cent lower risk of having depression.

St. John's Wort

St. John's wort (Hypericum perforatum) is a form of herbal mixture grown cure. It is viewed as a first-line antidepressant drug in some European nations. It is used for treatment for mild and moderate indications of depression, however, it has not been proven efficient in treating major depressive episodes.

St. John's wort may work like SSRIs. The regular dose is 300 mg 3 times each day with meals to forestall GI upset. On the off chance that no clinical reaction happens following 3–6 months, the use of another drug is suggested.

It is being considered as an alternative therapy for depression. The 2011 APA rule noticed that St. John's wort may be thought of, but evidence for its potency is developing, and more data is required about its interaction with other drugs.

Remember that positive changes in your exercise, everyday diet and sleep can make a big difference. These are the three things that are interconnected. They are essential when it comes to relaxing your body and soul.

You need to have lots of exercises which can help you sleep much better. You need to drink enough water as much water as you need. You ought to have completely balanced diets and highly nutritious meals. Try to include lots of fruits, greens and whole grains in your everyday diet.

The trio combination of exercise, daily balanced diet and sleep can truly have a major effect. These are the three things that are interconnected. They are an integral part of relaxing the body, mind and soul. You need to have an exercise which can assist you in sleeping better. Additionally, you can drink as much water as you need. Having decent eating habits and highly nourishing meals. Taking a lot of fruits, greens and whole grains regularly in your diet.

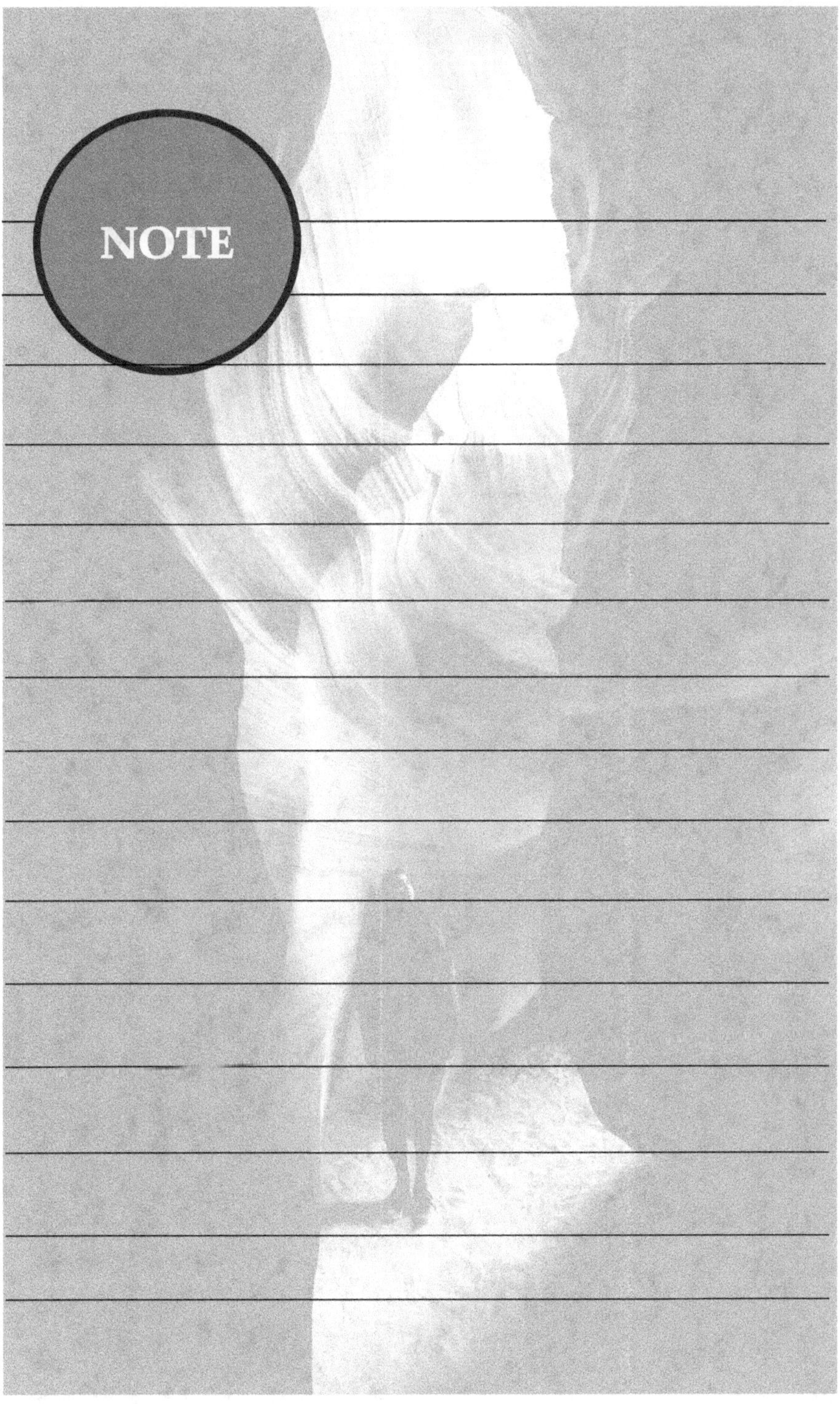

NOTE

Chapter Ten

Faith based approach to treatment of depression

Though the fig tree may not blossom, Nor fruit be on the vines; Though the labor of the live may fail, And the fields yield no food; Though the flock may be cut off from the fold, And there be no herd in the stalls. Yet I will rejoice in the LORD,
I will joy in the God of my salvation.

Chapter 10

FAITH BASED APPROACH TO TREATMENT OF DEPRESSION

Are you a Christian and are depressed? How does it feel? Your response and feelings may be feelings of being forgotten. Why you feeling so lonely and no one seems to be coming to your aid or understands you? You may even have the thought of challenging God; questions like "God where are you'? This could be what occupies your mind. After all, God said never will He leave you and never will He forsake you. Why then this rejection or loneliness with confusion shrouding you?

An encounter with a female student of mine's experience may put your present feelings in a better perspective; she emphatically told me that God has given up on her, so she is also giving up on God. She stopped attending church services. But, thank God, after counseling sessions with her, she found purpose in God again. In life, there are moments that seem we are in a dark tunnel struggling to come out with no hope at sight. Virtually everyone can experience depression. Even clerics do experiences depression. Some go to the extent of committing suicide. So, men of God are not shielded from this; the likes of Martin Luther and Ignatius de Loyola among others were not exempted. Even, Jesus Christ, our Lord, had his own dark moment, Isaiah 53: 2- 6. He had moment he was forsaken by friends, disciples, even his father (God) couldn't behold seeing him with the burden of human sins. At that point in his life he cried out depressed, saying, my God, my God why have you forsaken me?

But at the end of the tunnel there is light and Jesus was glorified. This session put in place critical measure that can help alleviate the impact of depression in you, only if you will submit yourself unto God.

Prayer therapy

The lyrics of a song many Christians sing tell the importance of prayer. Prayer is the master key to asking from God. Most times, we are full of grieves and can't think straight, we even take off the option of prayer during depression. Prayer is a great tool in walking with God in your darkest time. God is always closer to us in times of our troubles, because, Jesus had also experienced what you are passing through, so, He wants you to share with Him your experience of grief in prayer.

Prayer is a deliberate conversation or communing with God. Jesus said that anything we want we should ask in His name, including being delivered from depression, you can be healed of it. Prayer is a relational experience with the divine (God).

It is in our darkest moments that His light will shine. It is at this deepest moment if we cry unto God that He will come to our rescue. The lyric of the song mentioned earlier says:

First stanza: **What a friend we have in Jesus,**
All our sins and grieves he bears
What a privilege to carry
Everything to God in prayer!
O what peace we often forfeit
O what needless pain we bear,
All because we do not carry
Everything to God in prayer!

Second stanza: Have we trials and temptations!
Is there trouble anywhere?
We should never be discouraged

**Take it to the Lord in prayer.
Can we find a friend so faithful?
Who will all our sorrows share?
Jesus knows our every weakness:
Take it to the Lord in prayer.**

**Third stanza: Are we weak and heavy- laden,
Cumbered with a load of care
Precious Saviour, still our refuge
Take it to the Lord in prayer.
Do thy friends despise, forsake thee?
Take it to the Lord in prayer;
In His arms He'll take and shield thee,
Thou wilt find a solace there.**

Thus, stop complaining, you can talk to God in prayers.

Albeit, if at all you don't know what to say in the place of prayer, just cry unto God. He will help you to overcome just as Jesus came out of the darkest moment in His life gloriously.

Christian fellowship

Depression is easily known with loneliness and grief. Do you know that being involved and dedicated to the things of God can help reduce your chances of having depression? Little wonder this admonitions become paramount. "Let us not neglect meeting together, as it is the …" It is also a worthy saying that, "Iron sharpens iron," "two are better than one." The Christian life is symbolized with the cross. This shows an upward relationship with God in prayers as well as meditation in the word and sideward relationship with men. The bible says, make every efforts to live in peace with all men … These shows that no Christian (nobody) should live as an island.

Australian 10th Annual Suicide Prevention National Conference report by Larson shows that individuals who participated in religious gatherings and are serious about their faith have a low chance of having depressive disorder while people with less or low religious affinity have higher risk of major depression by 60%. Lack of organizational religious involvement is rated 20 - 60% increase in the numbers of individuals experiencing a major depressive episode.

At the end of the study, those who have ranked their religious faith as very important recover faster from their depression.

Having a religious faith is certainly important Valuing one's religious faith and identifying with them have importance and actively act as a social network group that can help to guard against depression. Members of such group tends to be closer to one another; share some heart-touching moment with a trusted ally. Or having something meaning set out as goals to achieve, the 'We'

feelings make an individual feels important about

his/her life thereby finding purpose for living.

However, not everyone in religious gathering is worthy

of sharing your deepest moment with.

Forgiveness therapy

Forgiveness is the act of letting go from your heart; to

pardon or having mercy on someone even when you

have been hurt. Forgiveness is one if the hardest

principles in Jesus' teachings, He commanded His

followers to forgive. In the Lord's Prayer, "And forgive

us our debts (wrongs), as we forgive our debtors (the

wrongs that others have done to us.)" This is an

injunction that is based on condition which depends on

us to accept or do otherwise.

Everyone wants to massage his or egos, wants justice, feel the memories and pains of uneventful incidence in order to express how we feel. But one thing I know about unforgiveness is that, it always comes with bitterness and grief. Since forgiveness is a hard choice we must learn to forgive by faith.

While you have genuine reasons you will not forgive, these reasons bring about retaining and withholding negative emotions such as grief, hatred, anger and darkness in your mind.

When I was younger, back in the days in secondary school, I had a friend who I kept malice with. I noticed that when I am with my other friends I felt okay and happy. Many adjudged me very lively, but the moment my friend passes by, my mood changes, I felt the hurt for over four years. My mood and countenance changed like that of the "Angry Bird".

I walked up to my friend one day and told her how I have been feeling towards her in recent years, "but I have forgiven you for Christ's sake", I said to her. But in reality, it's for my sake not; for my peace of mind, emotion and straight thinking.

Unforgiveness leads to retaining and withholding you as prisoner to grief, anger, hurt, and wanting to revenge. Forgiveness brings peace and joy to your emotion. For me, I didn't realize it until I told my friend whom I thought had offended me. She said, "Sam, I never knew you were hurt by my actions. I am sorry." So, the negative emotions I have borne all these years did not affect her. What a prisoner of unforgiveness I was!

When you forgive you let go off you negative feelings, thereby letting go of the anger and hurt and ultimately a way of improving your health and immune system. Studies have shown that individuals with feelings of anger and hurt tend to have poor health and prone to chronic illness, depression is not left out. There is a great increase in the level of the stress, hormone cortisol that suppresses the system.

When we forgiveness others their wrong doings we do ourselves a great deal of physical, social and spiritual goodness.

Forgiveness is not what you just profess, it is a thing of the mind. Your forgiveness is tested when you see the cause of your unforgiveness and do not feel hurt. I have seen my friend over and over again. And each time we see, I felt I had been a prisoner to my friend who psychologically controlled my emotions. However, Jesus said forgiveness is continuous thing we do every time.

Jesus' disciple Peter once came to Jesus and asked, "Lord, if my brother keeps on sinning against me, how many times do I have to forgive him? Seven times?" "No, not seven times," answered Jesus, "but seventy times seven.

Unforgiveness imprisons you, your attitudes and thoughts.

The tightened palm

From the above, it is easier to say that forgiveness is a hard choice every Christian must make. This was exactly my response to the student of mine. She lamented that she had been sexually abused by her

Uncle's son. She was scared of going back to her village, as a result she kept it to herself for years, until it became unbearable any longer. There was a particular day, after the school she attended had closed for the day, which she couldn't go home because of the molestation, harassment and physical assaults being melted on her by her cousin. It dawned on the relatives when they noticed that it was getting dark and the physically matured teenager was not back home from school. They came to the school to know what have kept her back. They were shocked when they realized that she was also not in the school. After much ado which brought both the family and the school management together, they found her in a classmate's house. There, she told the reason for her action. She was entreated and taken back home.

One day, after my allotted teaching time had elapsed, she called my attention to her mood. She accused me of not being sensitive enough about her mood, and that she was struggling to understand anything being taught in the school because majority of the school teachers were men. She said any time anyone taught her she saw the reflections of her cousin who was assaulting her and brought back the deadly moment she have had.

I understood her enough that she was trying to share a burden with me. I listened to her pathetic story and got closer to her. She told me that she had less believe in God; she doesn't attend church, no friends but only friends in school, and home experience is like a prison and she was not ready to leave the city, hence, the reason for her endurance.

Having listened to her, and being closer, I told her that she should consider forgiving everyone who have offended her including her cousin. She became emotional. I told her to give me her hand. I looked into her wet eyes and palm as I later folded the palm.

After a few minutes heat had generated in the folded palm, as a result she became uncomfortable. Then, I told her that her unforgiveness is likened to the heat being generated in her palm, and that she had to open it up and let go so that she can enjoy fresh air in the palm. But in the process folding the palm she felt and saw the pains and anguish; memories of the past which hunt her. She was at a point unwilling to forgive and the palm remained closed. But later, she opened up her palm and felt the freedom. I told her that opening up of her palm is an expression showing that she can't help herself and opened up unto God as a way of surrendering herself unto God to come and help her. But without letting go, and opening up the palm God cannot come in because her palm is tight.

So, open up the palm of your heart and let the Lord help you through your grief and hunting memories. Jesus said come unto me all you who are labored and heavy ladened, I will give you rest.

My student has since forgiven and found purpose for living. She wants to be a legal practitioner so that she can speak for anyone in similar situation. No more suicidal thoughts; and she has found rest for her soul in Christ.

Job's lesson: overcoming loss

Anguish and depression are two related yet different reactions that are confusedly understood to be the same. Anguish is the body's ordinary reaction to a misfortune and loss. In the wake of encountering a major loss, some individuals experience a serious loss, this bring about great sense of emotion and physical response. The vast majority of people easily adjust to the reality of the demise or loss of a beloved. With time, the lamenting individual learns to acclimate to their life that has been changed by the death or loss. At the point when the typical grief reaction doesn't improve about a month after the loss and the situation deteriorate almost consistently, concerns ought to be raised, the situation may result into a clinical depression.

The life of Job ought to be a consolation to Christians during the loss of their loved ones. This infers that you are only a manager of God's creations in this world not the proprietor or owner, thus, the real owner can make demand of what you think you have. When you are faced with loss, you ought to consider it as returning what you have been trusted with to your Lord. So we read from Job that after his children and riches were all destroyed in one day, he got up and tore his garments in grief. He shaved his head and hurled himself faced bowed to the ground. He said, "I was born with nothing, and I will die with nothing. The Lord gave, and now he has taken away."

In the wake of encountering such a significant misfortune, Job did show serious despondency and depressive signs, rather, He contended with his companions (friends, maybe not his wife) and God in questioning for what has happened to him. Through the process, he got healed and got over the depressive mood.

This kind of Christian faith encourages one to adapt to the loss of the parted beloved by letting go of it. Of course, past memories of the deceased may linger on in our minds, but we must learn to let it go. This disposition helps in reducing the danger of forming into complicated situation, such as clinical depression. For the Christian, making claim of having nothing doesn't imply that you don't have anything. Jesus told his disciples that, "If any of you want to come with me, you must forget yourself, carry your cross, and follow me.

Take charge of your thought

The mind of man is said to be the seat of knowledge; good and evil emanates from the mind (heart). Events in life are receptive based on how the mind perceives them. The Bible teaches, anyone who accept Jesus Christ becomes a child of God, as such, his/her is given a new mind. And having a new mind means a lot in Christendom. The Bible says that "we have the mind of Christ." This kind of mind is not sense based (what you see, feel, taste, hear, smell), but faith based; 'for we walk by faith not by sight."

The bible admonishes that, 'And do not be conformed to this world, but be transformed by the renewing of your mind, that you may prove what *is* that good and acceptable and perfect will of God.' Your mind matters a lot in your times of tribulation, grief or depression. Having a mind of Christ will help you in collaboration with your Christian partners to see God in what you pass through.

Do not allow what you are passing through define you. Don't let grief, pains, disappointment, loss of a beloved, job, friend, relationship etc. define who you are, they are mere events in life, but, be transformed in your mind. What you think about yourself have a way of manifestation in reality. "For as he thinks in his heart, so *is* he."

The good news is that there are many testimonies of individuals who have recovered from depression, anxiety, fear and other mental health issues, yours won't be an exception. Think well about yourself and you will have it.

The more time you spend reading and thinking about His Word, the more it gets inside of you and begins to change you from the inside out. Hebrews 4:12 says that God's Word "is alive and powerful".

Biblical Prescription for Depression

Depression may be as a result of a physical or chemical imbalance, this may not be disputable, and however, some individuals may find themselves having depression as a result of spiritual issues. Here are a few bible verses that give instructions on how to fight depression.

Bible Verses about Depression

Ps 30:11: *You have turned for me my mourning into dancing; you have put off my sackcloth and clothed me with gladness*, NKJV

Ps 3:3: *Butt You, O L*ORD*, are a shield for me, my glory and the One who lifts up my head.* NKJV

Deut. 31:8: *And the L*ORD*, He is the One who goes before you. He will be with you, He will not leave you nor forsake you; do not fear nor be dismayed."* NKJV

Isa 40:31: *But those who wait on the L*ORD *shall renew their strength; they shall mount up with wings like eagles, they shall run and not be weary, they shall walk and not faint.* NKJV

John 10:10: *The thief does not come except to steal, and to kill, and to destroy. I have come that they may have life, and that they may have it more abundantly.* NKJV

Phil 4:13: *I can do all things through Christ* who strengthens me.* NKJV

John 16:33: *These things I have spoken to you, that in Me you may have peace. In the world you will* have*

tribulation; but be of good cheer, I have overcome the world." NKJV

Scripture Quotes on Depression

Isa 41:10: *Fear not, for I am with you; Be not dismayed, for I am your God. I will strengthen you, Yes, I will help you, I will uphold you with My righteous right hand.'*

NKJV

Matt 11:28-29: *Come to Me, all you who labor and are heavy laden, and I will give you rest.* NKJV

Jer 29:11-12: *For I know the thoughts that I think toward you, says the LORD, thoughts of peace and not of evil, to give you a future and a hope.* NKJV

Prov 3:5: *Trust in the LORD with all your heart, and lean not on your own understanding; all your ways acknowledge Him, And He shall direct your paths.* NKJV

Ps 30:5: *For His anger is but for a moment, His favor is for life; Weeping may endure for a night, But joy comes in the morning.* NKJV

Depression Bible Verses

1 Peter 5:7: *Casting all your care upon Him, for He cares for you.*

Ps 143:7-8: *Answer me speedily, O LORD; My spirit fails! Do not hide Your face from me, Lest I be like those who go down into the pit. Cause me to hear Your loving-kindness in the morning, For in You do I trust; Cause me to know the way in which I should walk, For I lift up my soul to You.* NKJV

Phil 4:6: *Be anxious for nothing, but in everything by prayer and supplication, with thanksgiving, let your requests be made known to God;* NKJV

Ps 23:4: *Yea, though I walk through the valley of the shadow of death, I will fear no evil; For You are with me; Your rod and Your staff, they comfort me.* NKJV

Rom 8:28: *And we know that all things work together for good to those who love God, to those who are the called according to His purpose.* NKJV

Depression in the Bible

Prov 12:25: *Anxiety in the heart of man causes depression, But a good word makes it glad.* NKJV

Rom 12:2: *And do not be conformed to this world, but be transformed by the renewing of your mind, that you may prove what is that good and acceptable and perfect will of God.* NKJV

Ps 9:9: *The LORD also will be a refuge for the oppressed, A refuge in times of trouble.* NKJV

2 Tim 1:7: *For God has not given us a spirit of fear, but of power and of love and of a sound mind.*

Rev 21:4: *And God will wipe away every tear from their eyes; there shall be no more death, nor sorrow, nor crying. There shall be no more pain, for the former things have passed away."* NKJV

Bible Verses for When You're Depressed

Ps 34:17-18: *The righteous cry out, and the LORD hears, and delivers them out of all their troubles. The LORD is near to those who have a broken heart, and saves such as have a contrite spirit.* NKJV

Matthew 6:33: *But seek first the kingdom of God and his righteousness, and all these things will be added to you.* **ESV**

Romans 15:13: *May the God of hope fill you with all joy and peace in believing, so that by the power of the Holy Spirit you may abound in hope.* **ESV**

John 16:33: *I have said these things to you, that in me you may have peace. In the world you will have tribulation. But take heart; I have overcome the world.* *ESV*

Joshua 1:9: *Have I not commanded you? Be strong and courageous. Do not be frightened, and do not be dismayed, for the Lord your God is with you wherever you go."* **ESV**

183

Depression doesn t have to rule your life. No matter what you re going through, God is ready and willing to help you take your pain.. and turn it into something great.

Joyce Meyer

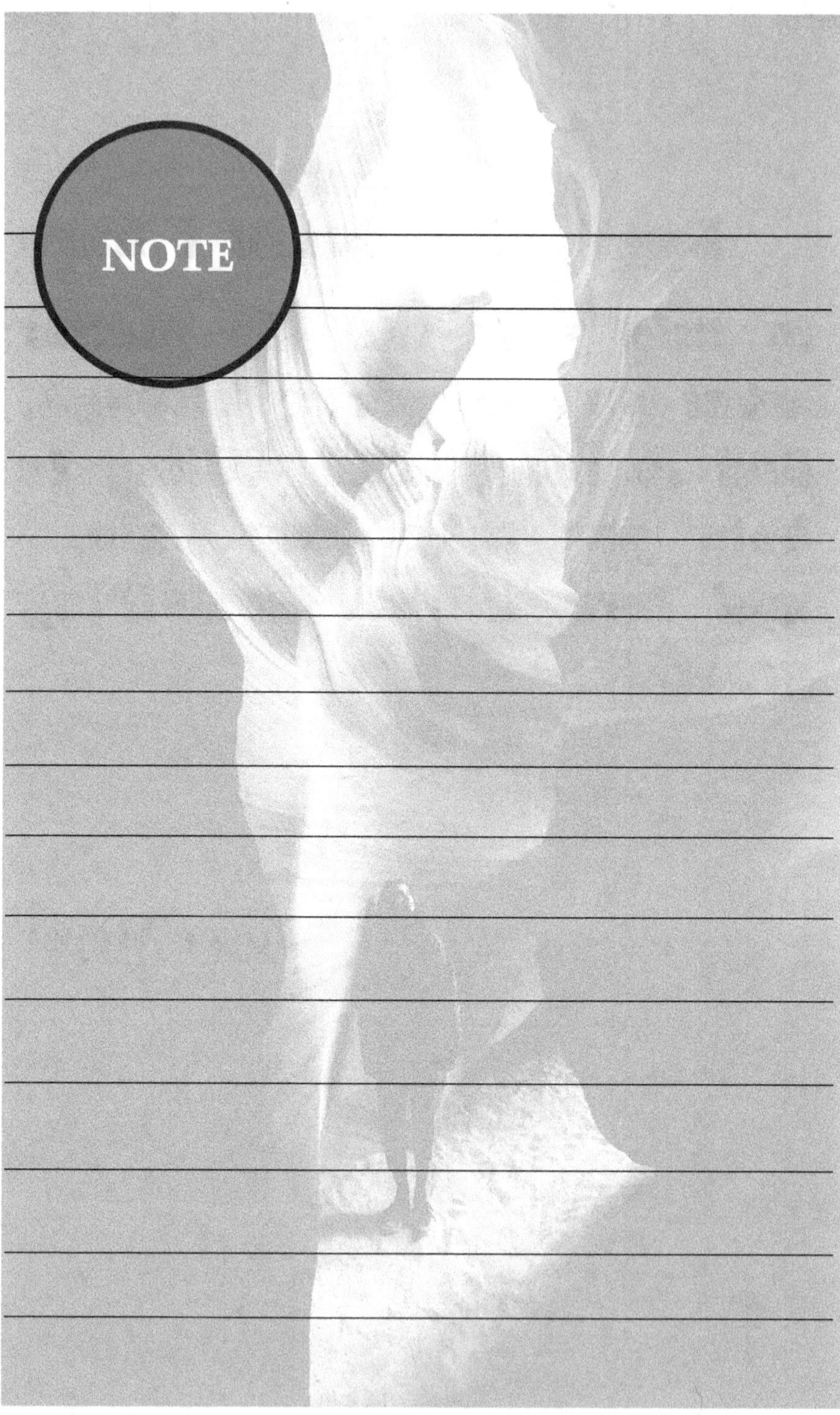
NOTE

About the *Author*

Sam Oluwaseyi is a multi-dimensional person, a writer, author, counsellor, educationist, publisher, jounalist and entrepreneur.

He has a Degree in Mass Communication. As a publisher, he has a monthly Christian publication known as The Sparklight Gospel Publications. The contributive positive imparts of his works have indelible marks in the minds of people. He knows that helping other to find their paths in life is what give him joy. He has a successful marriage.

Acknowledgments

Deepest gratitude to the Almight God for the success of this book. I appreciate my wife, Eunice, and Sam Ade (My teacher).s

THANKS FOR READING